100

Yoga Themed Puzzles

60 Yoga Themed Sudoku Puzzles
40 Yoga Themed Mazes

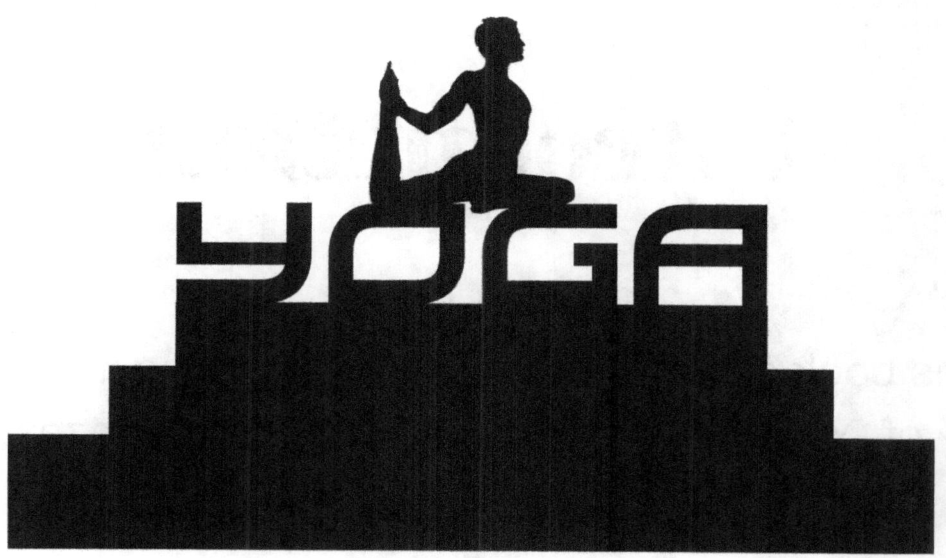

This
Yoga
Themed Puzzle
Book
Belongs To:

____

Introduction

This book consists of 60 Sudoku puzzles made up of Yoga themed images - **PLUS** 40 Mazes composed of Yoga images

Doing these puzzles is a great way to have a lot of fun, improve your focus, logic and problem solving abilities.

These puzzles are tough - but solvable! You are going to have a great time and get a lot of satisfaction out of working out the solutions.

Get ready for hours and hours of FUN!

Mazes
Instructions

These Mazes are very easy to understand but (at least some of them) are very HARD to actually do!

Personally, I've found that the mazes in most books are aimed at little kids and are so easy, they aren't worth the time... not these.

These Yoga themed, shaped mazes have four basic levels of difficulty. Easiest (not simple), Medium, Hard and OMG!

Each puzzle has a tiny little "S" somewhere... That indicates where to start - then there is a little "E" somewhere that indicates where to stop. Sometimes in the more complex puzzles, it is a challenge to even find the "S" and the "E" but take heart, they ARE there.

Sudoku Instructions

The standard Sudoku's objective is to fill a 9×9 grid with numbers so that each column, each row, and each of the nine 3×3 boxes that compose the main grid contain all of the digits from 1 to 9.

None of the digits can be repeated in the same row, column or 3x3 box.

USUALLY!

Sudoku puzzles are logic problems, not number problems. The 1 through 9 digits can be replaced by letters, symbols, words or even pictures... just so there are 9 unique characters to work with. **These puzzles** are made up of nine different Yoga themed images rather than numbers. The solving logic is the same as it would be if they were numbers, but using images adds an extra layer of fun.

To get you started, a few of the squares have already been filled in. The next page shows the nine images used in these puzzles. You can solve using the images - or - you can assign a number to each of them and solve the normal way.

Sudoku Image legend

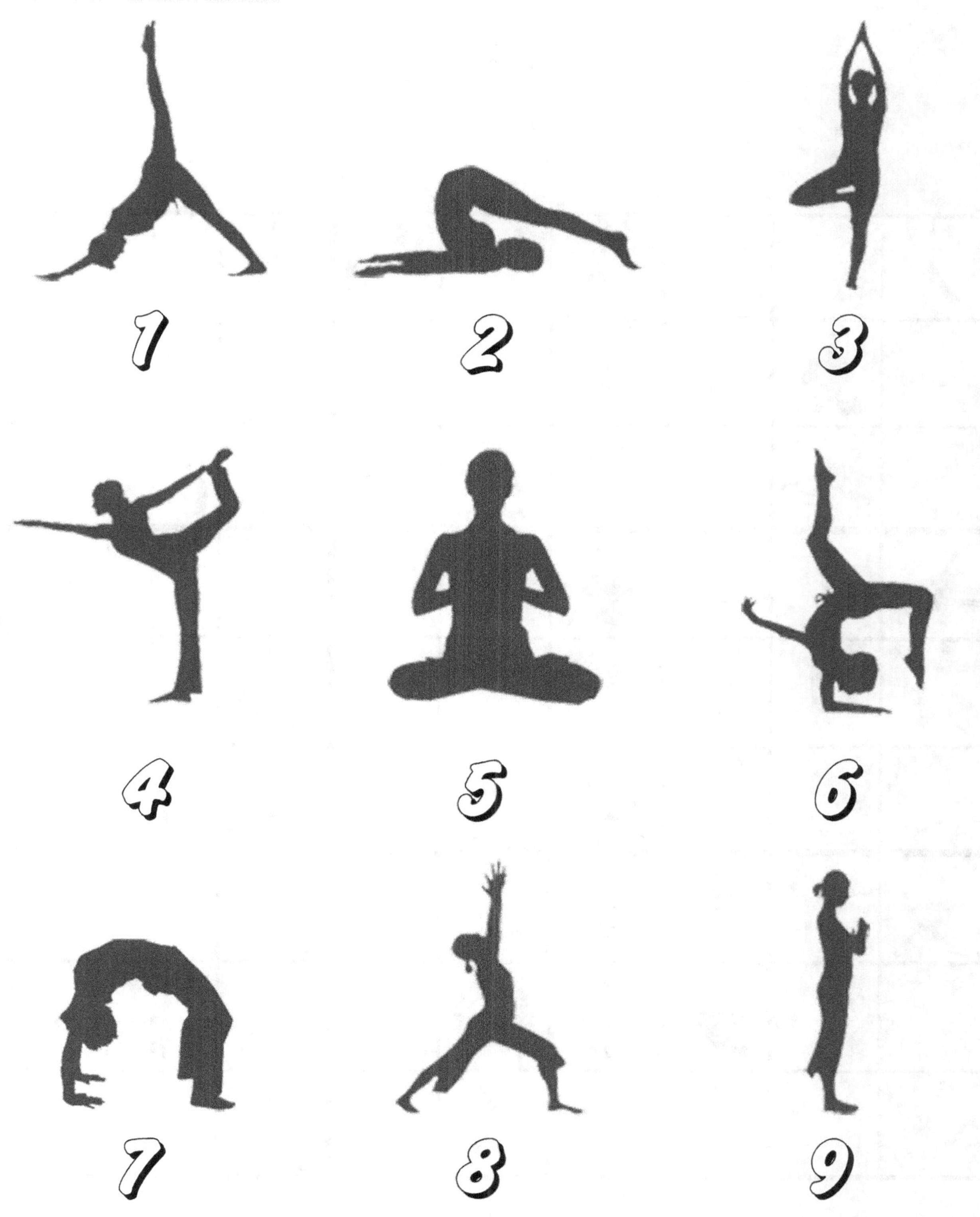

Sudoku #1

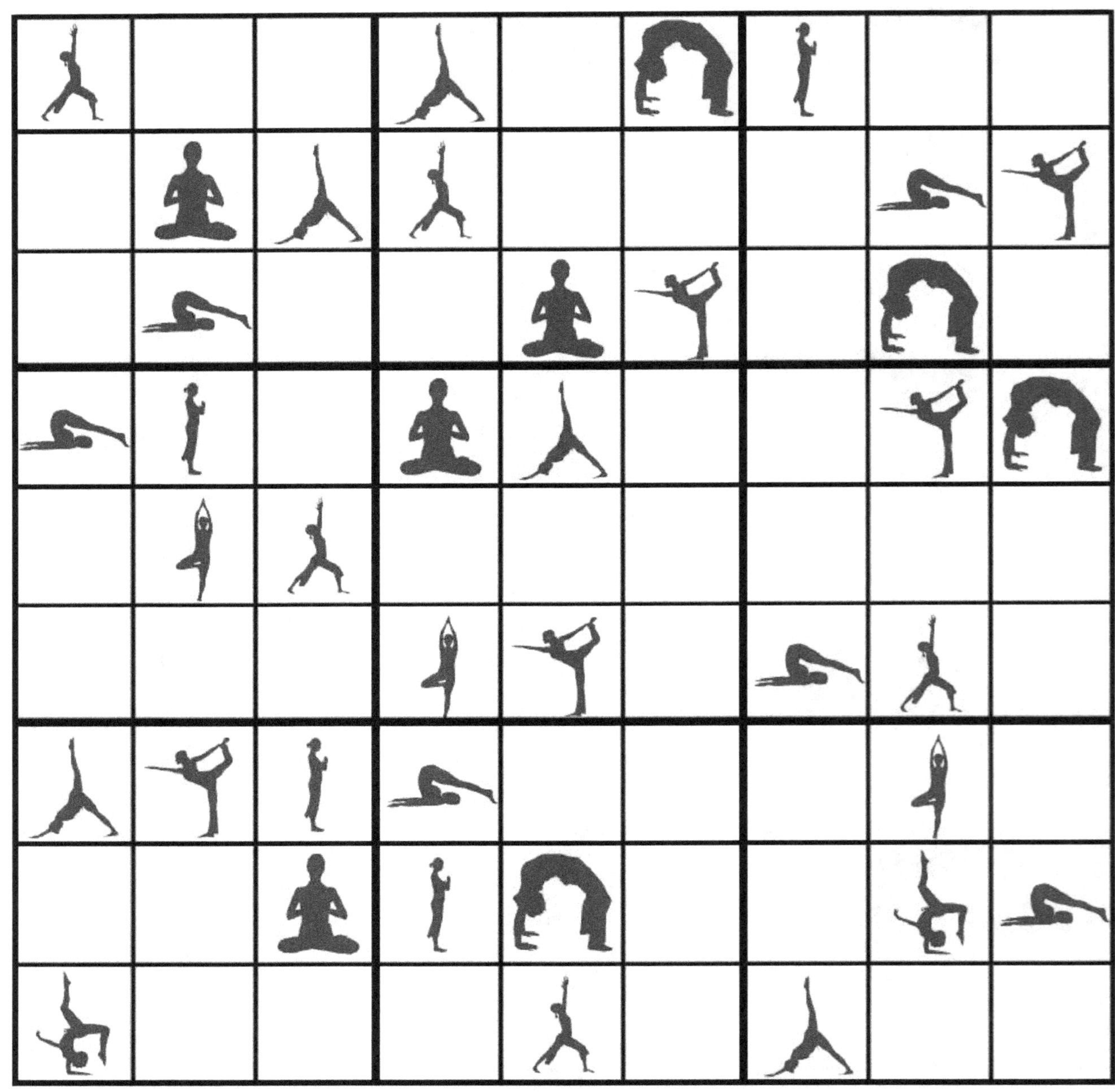

Yoga
Maze #1

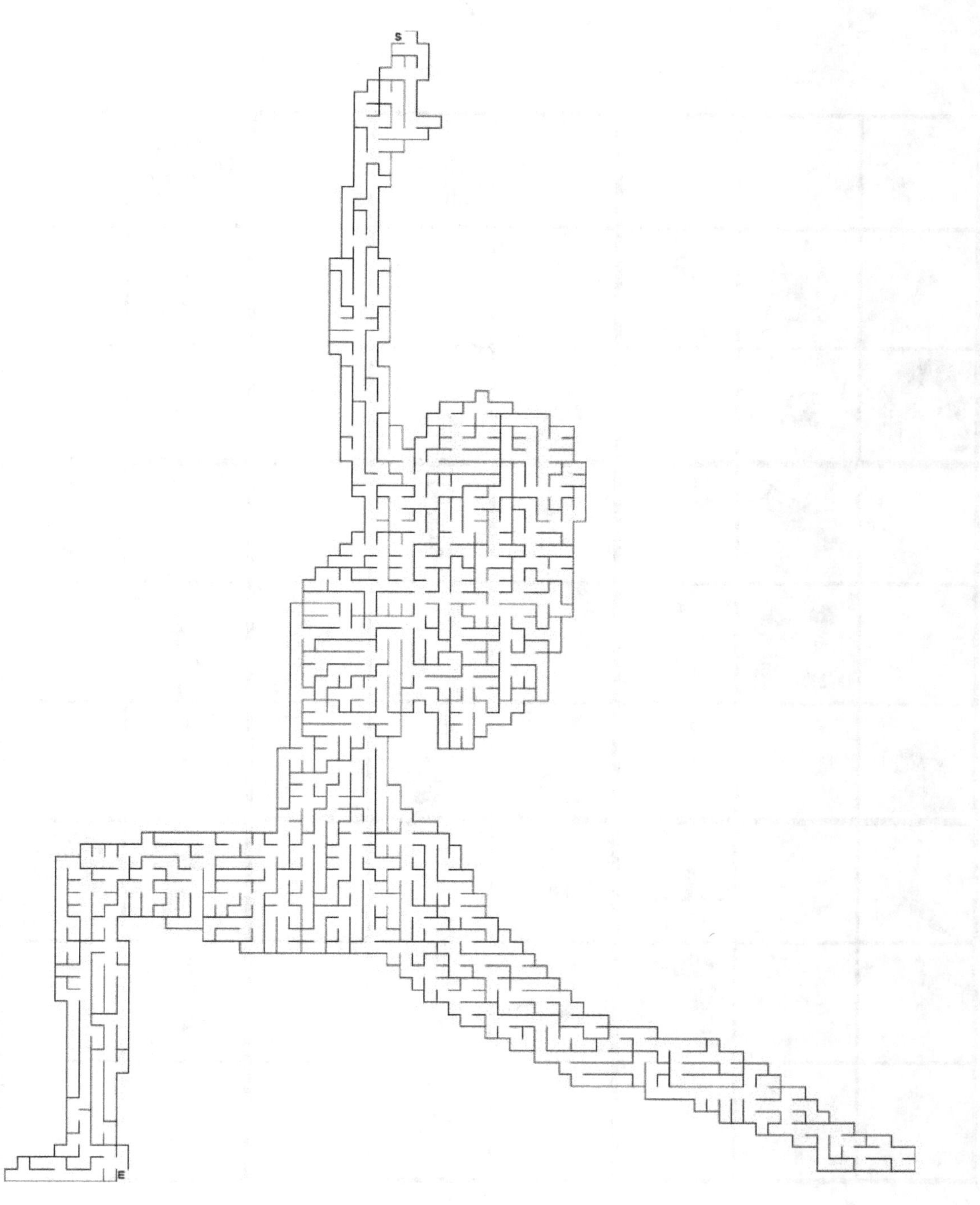

Sudoku #2

Yoga
Maze #2

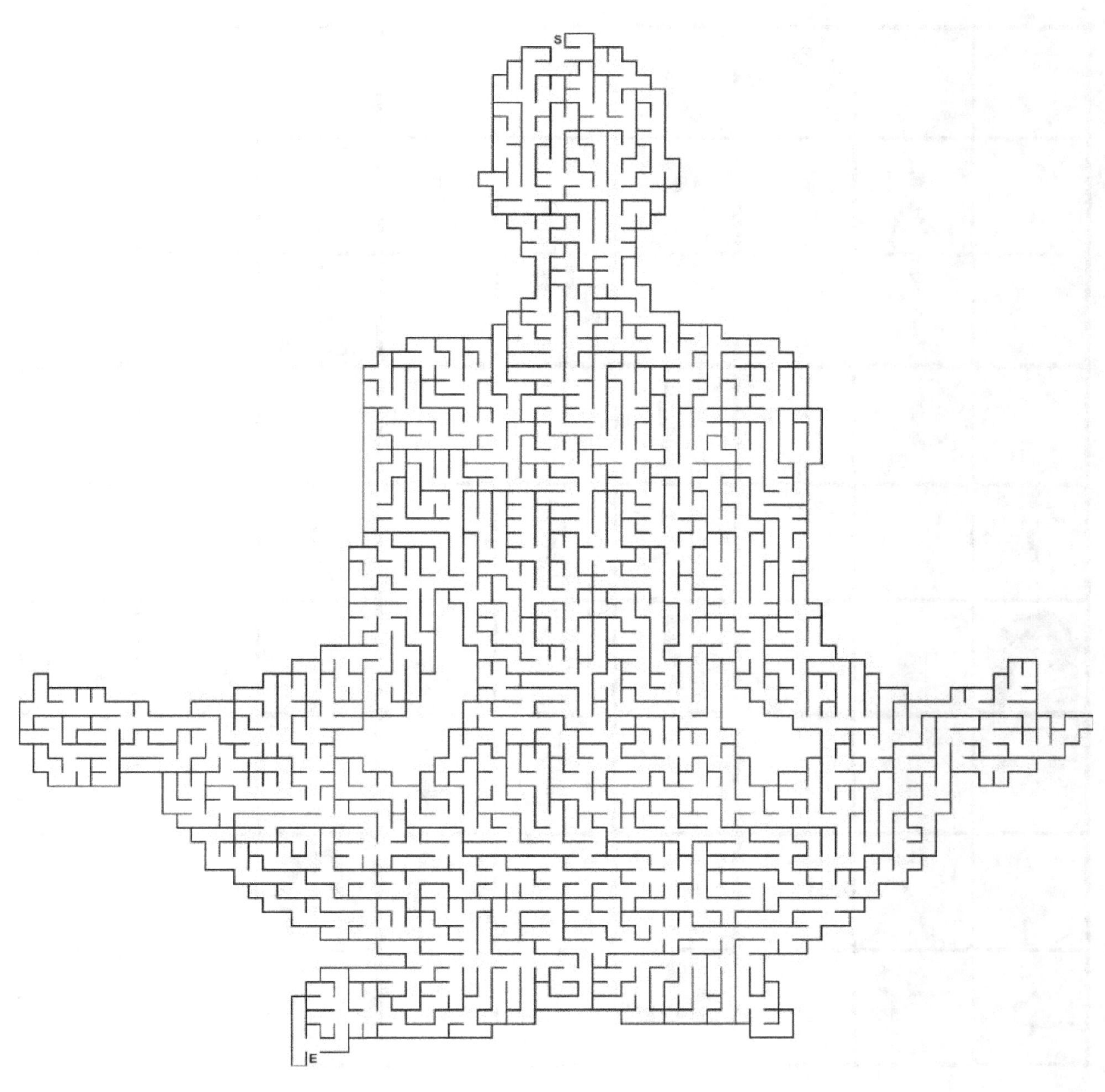

Sudoku #3

★

Yoga
Maze #3

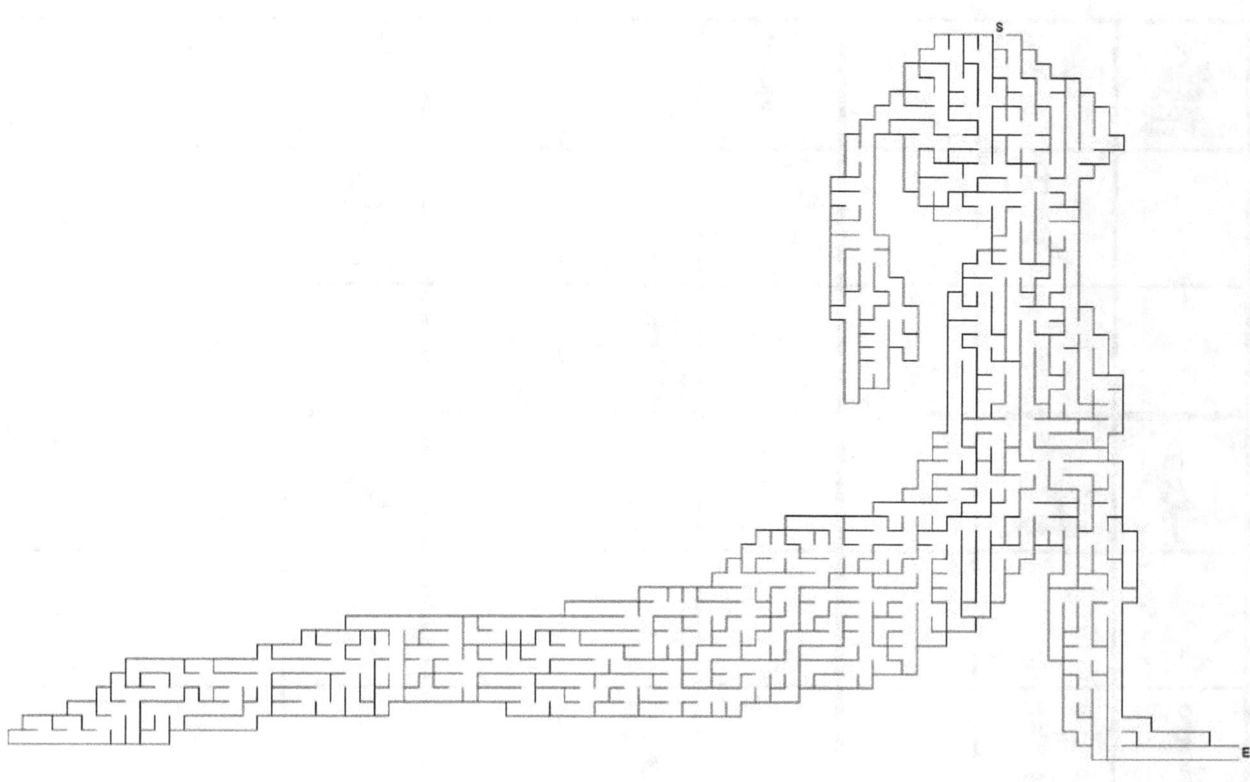

Sudoku #4

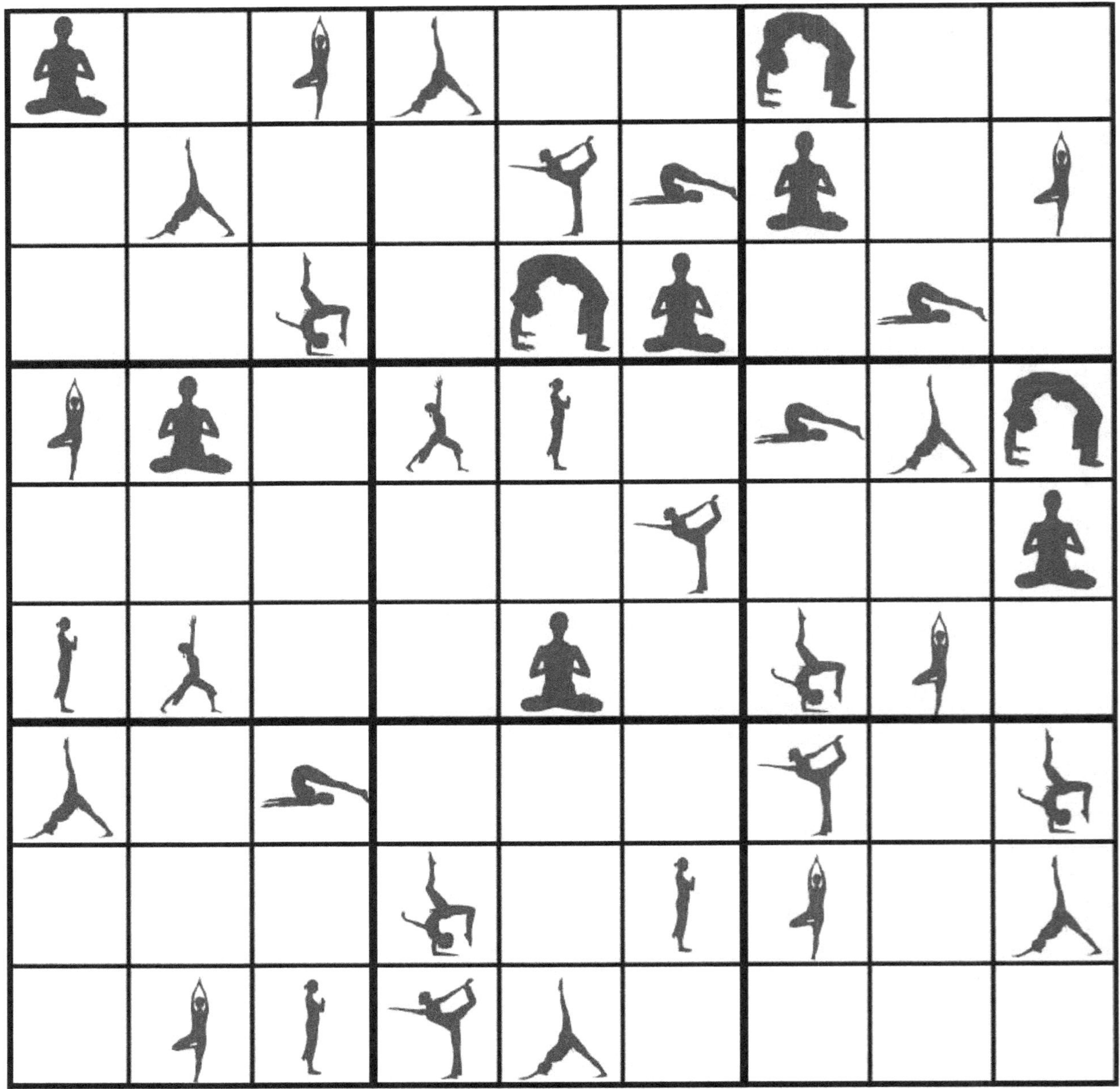

Yoga
Maze #4

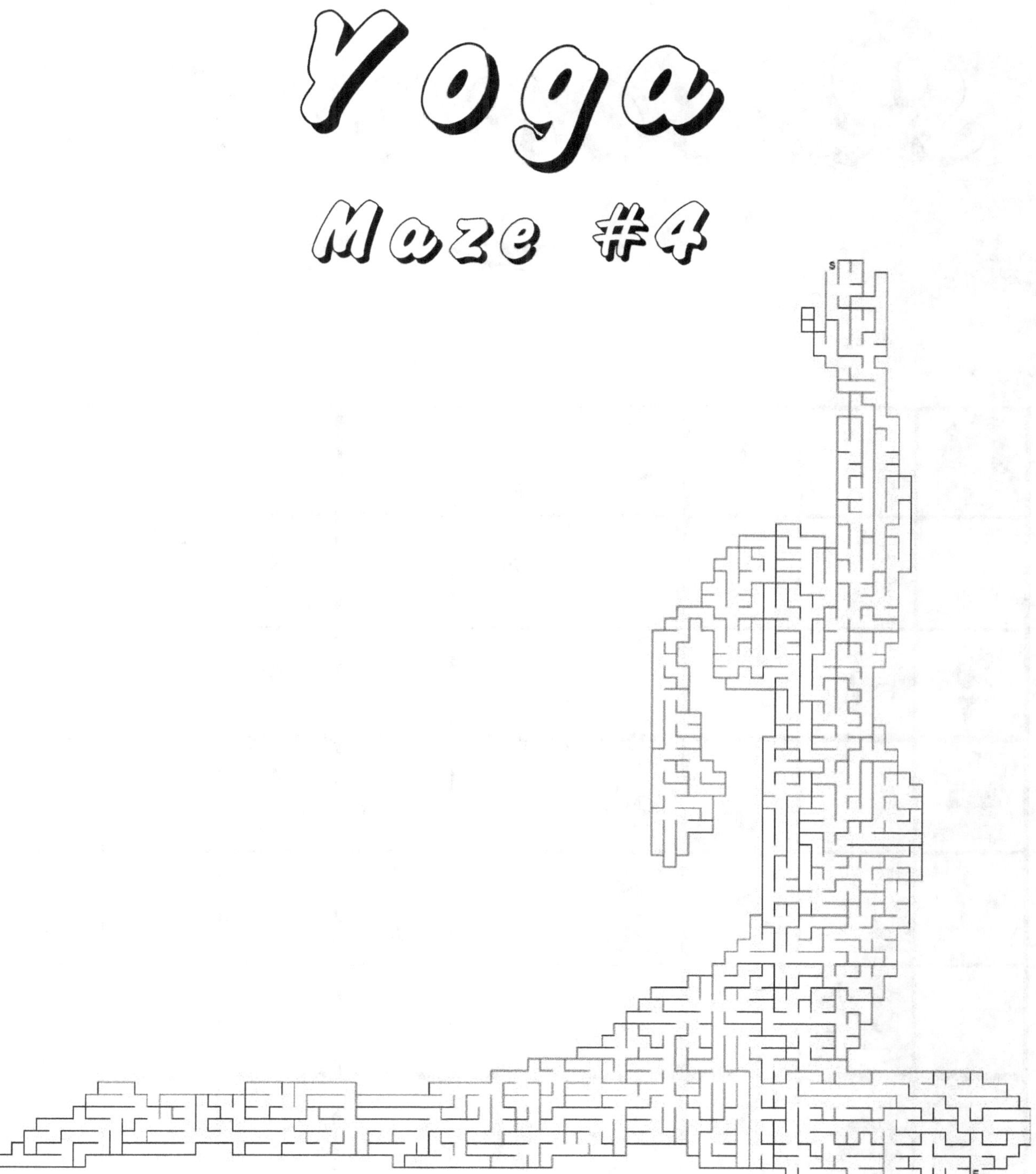

Sudoku #5

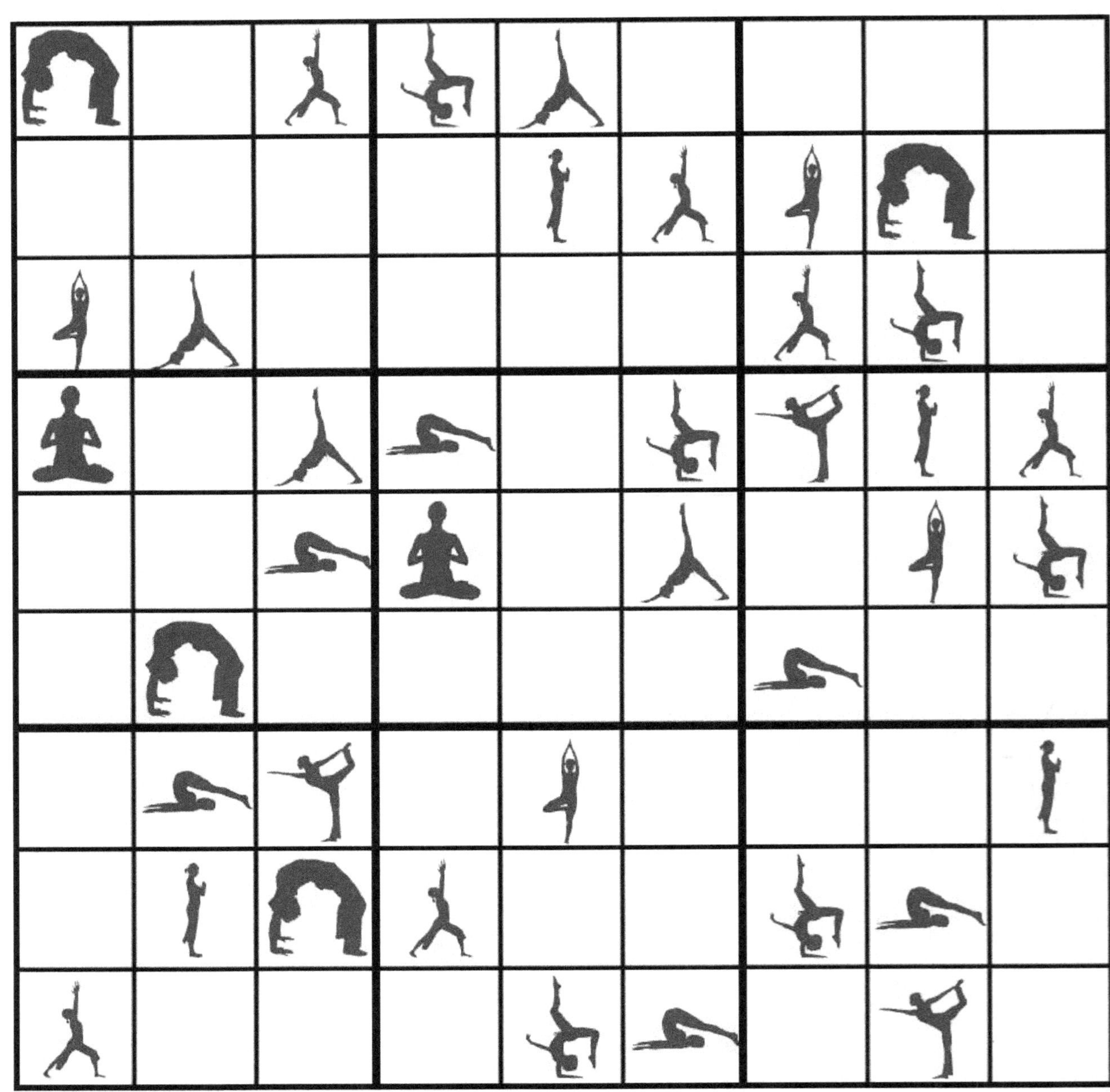

Yoga

Maze #5

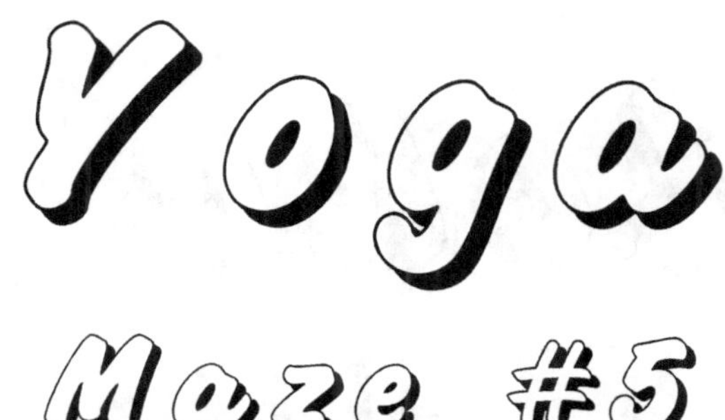

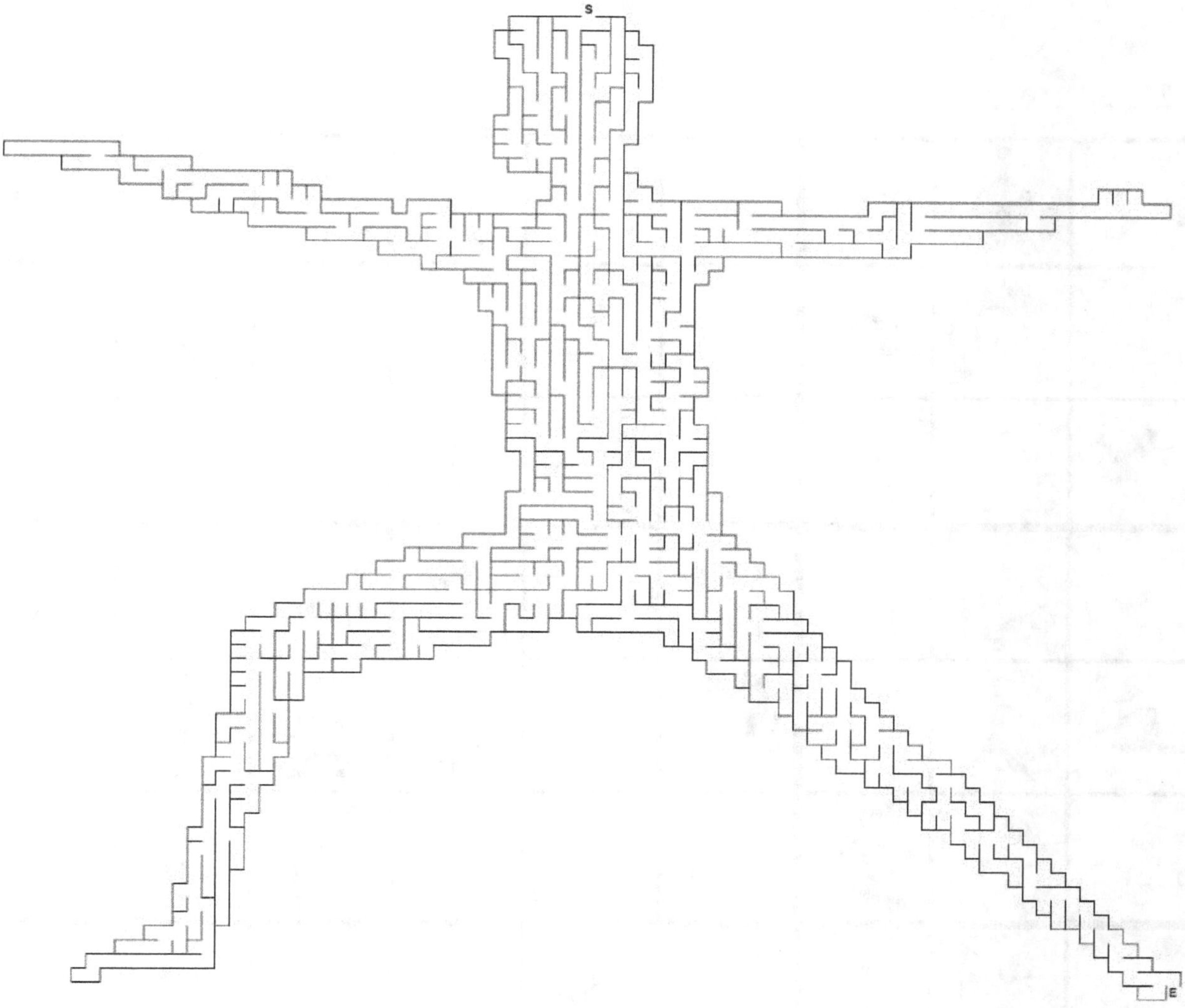

Sudoku #6

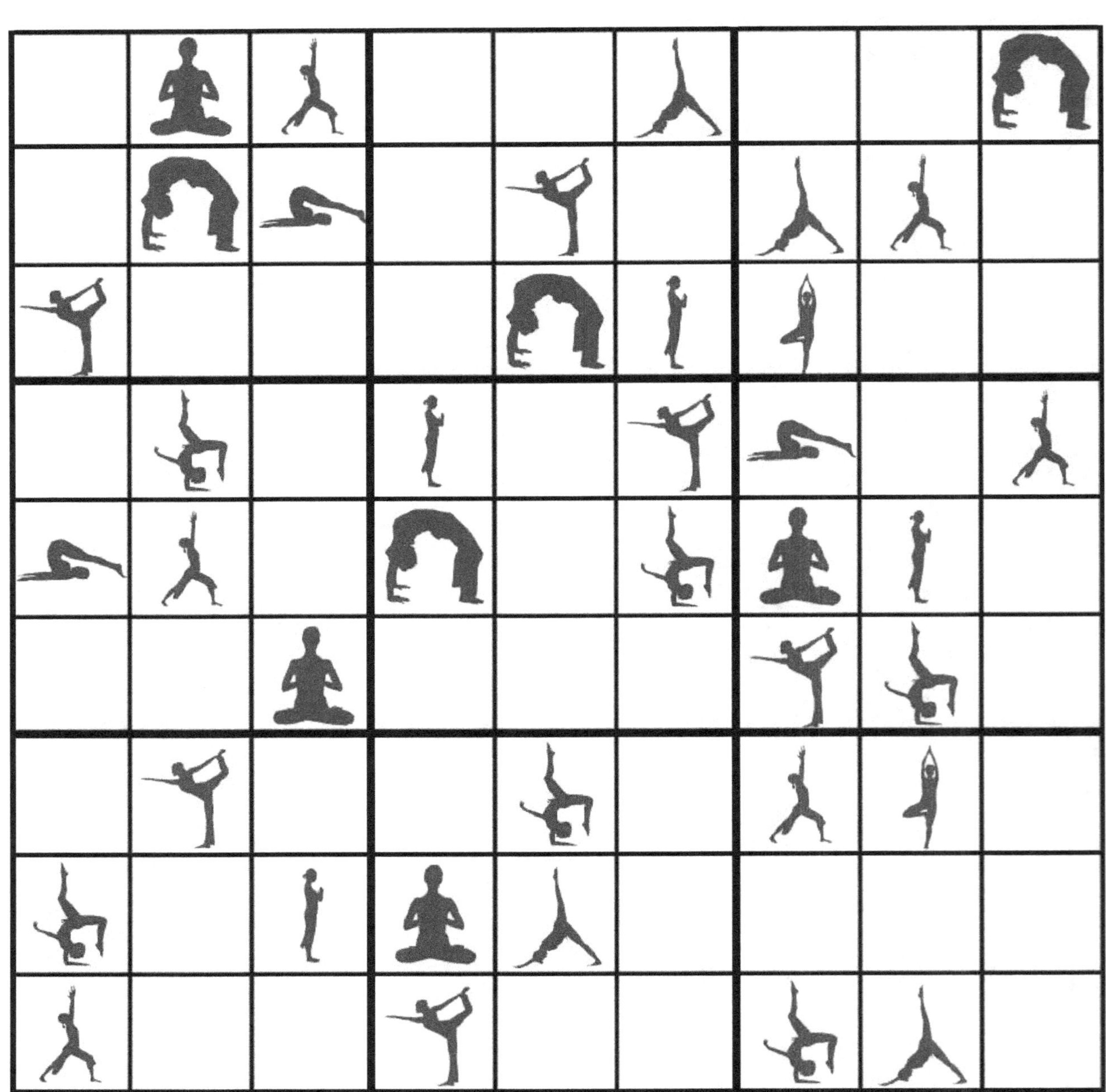

Yoga

Maze #6

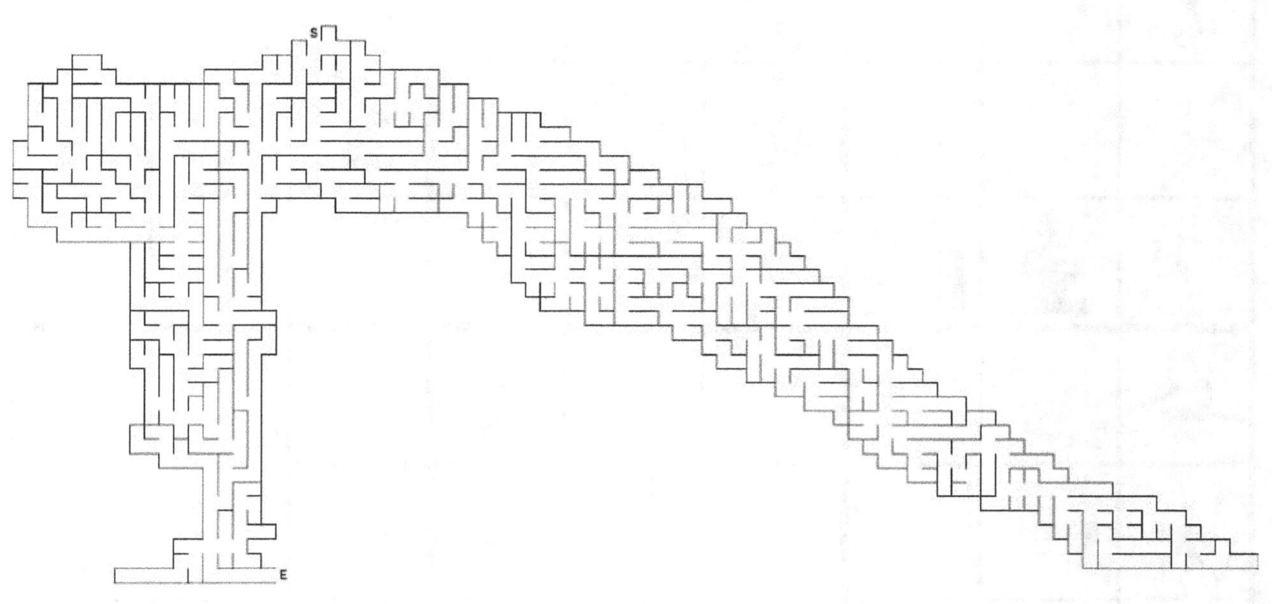

Sudoku #7

Yoga
Maze #7

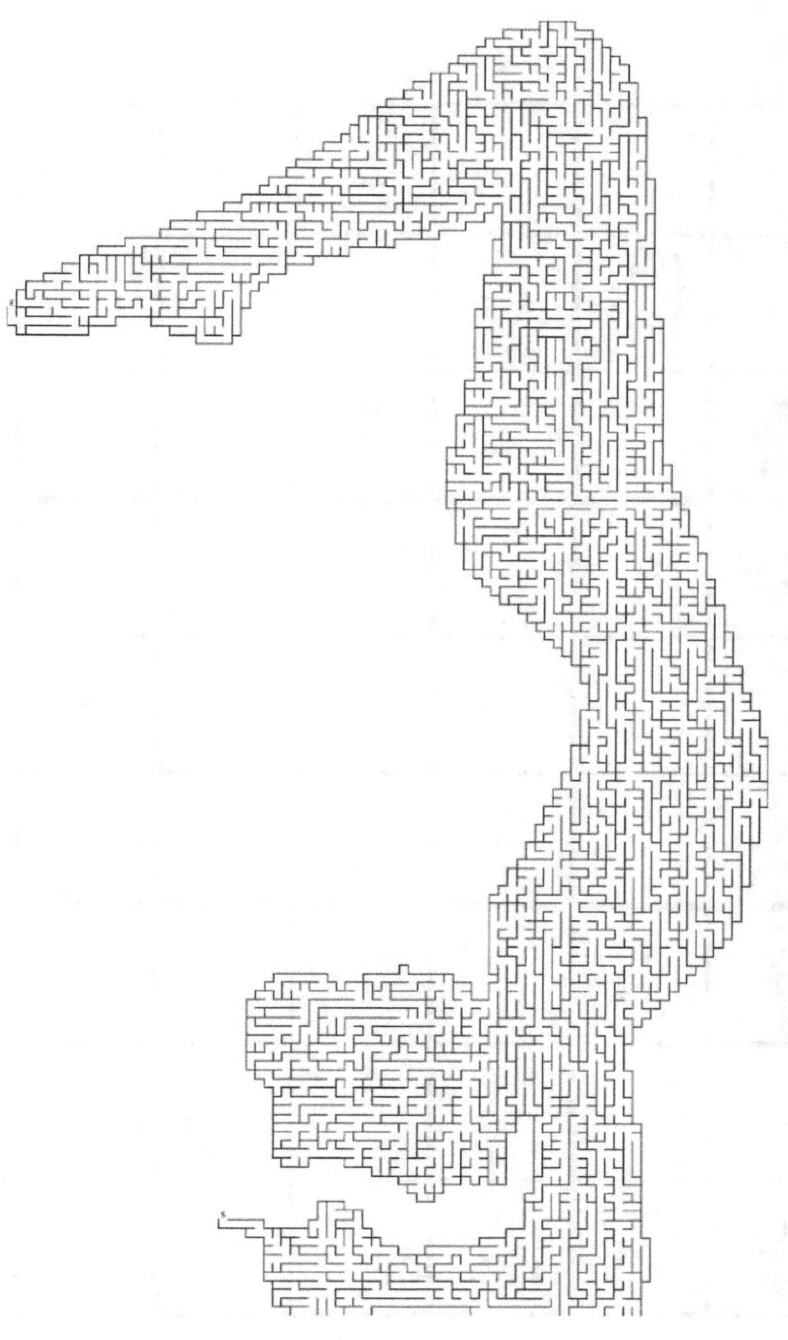

Sudoku #8

Yoga

Maze #8

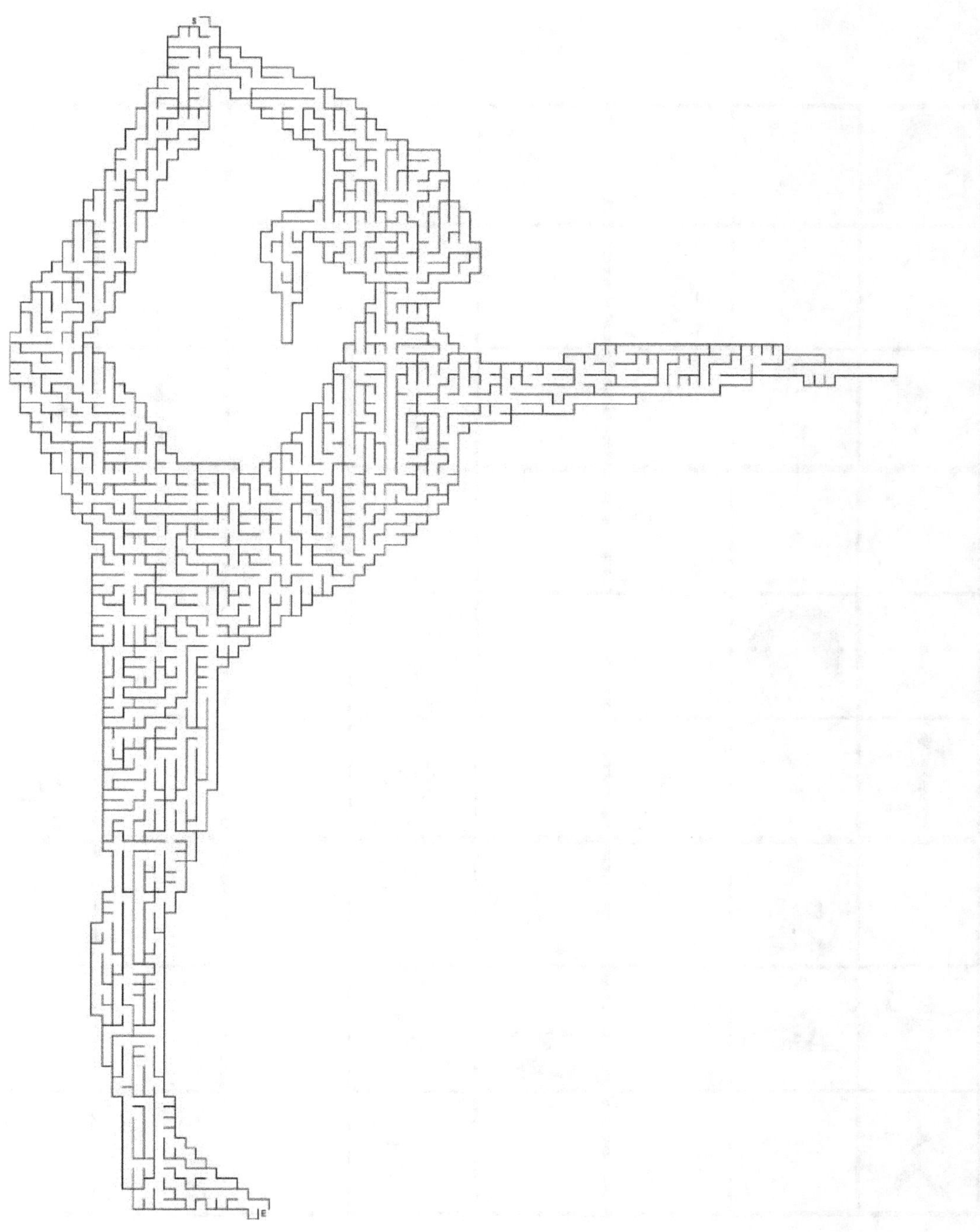

Sudoku #9

★

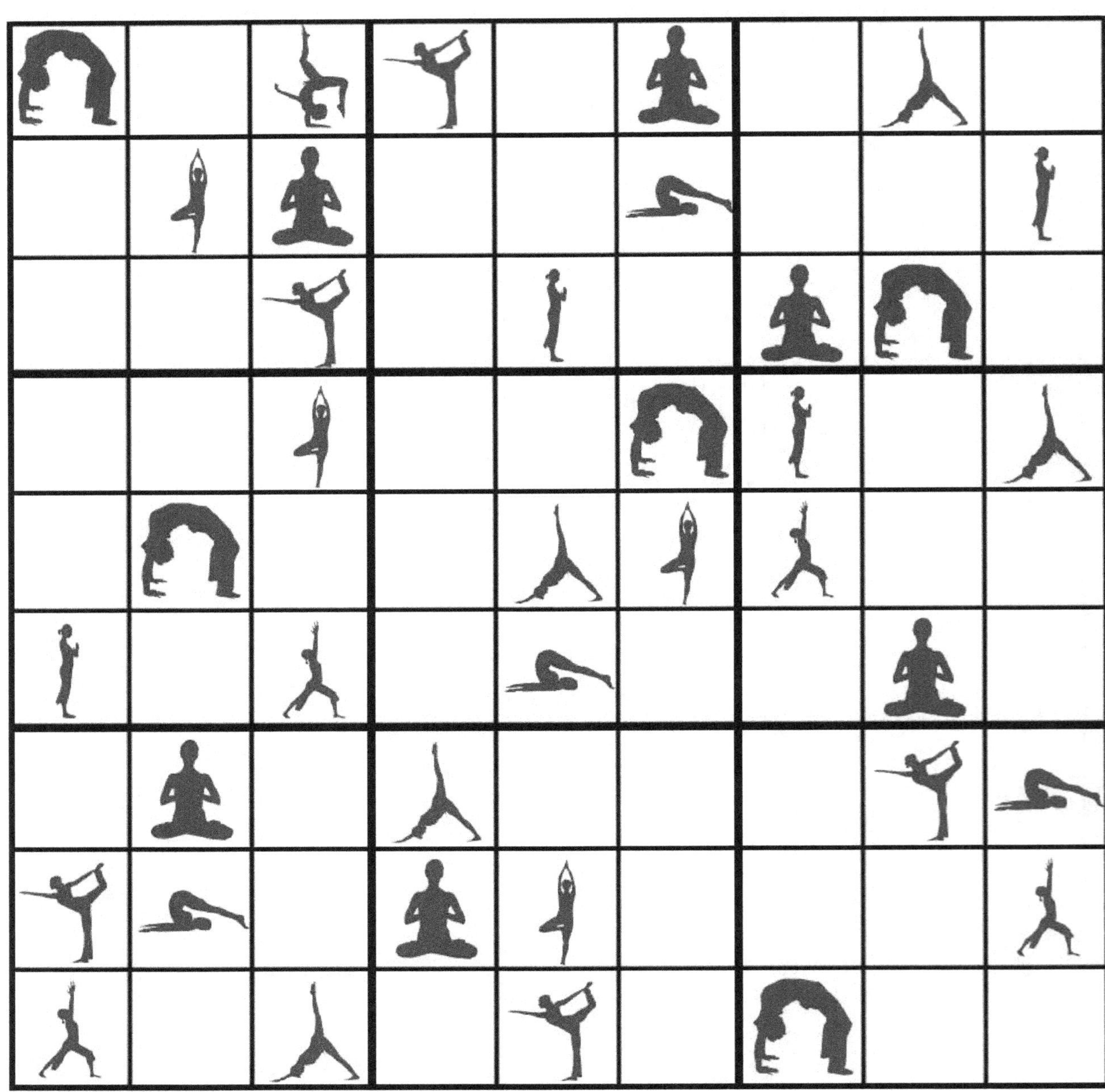

Yoga
Maze #9

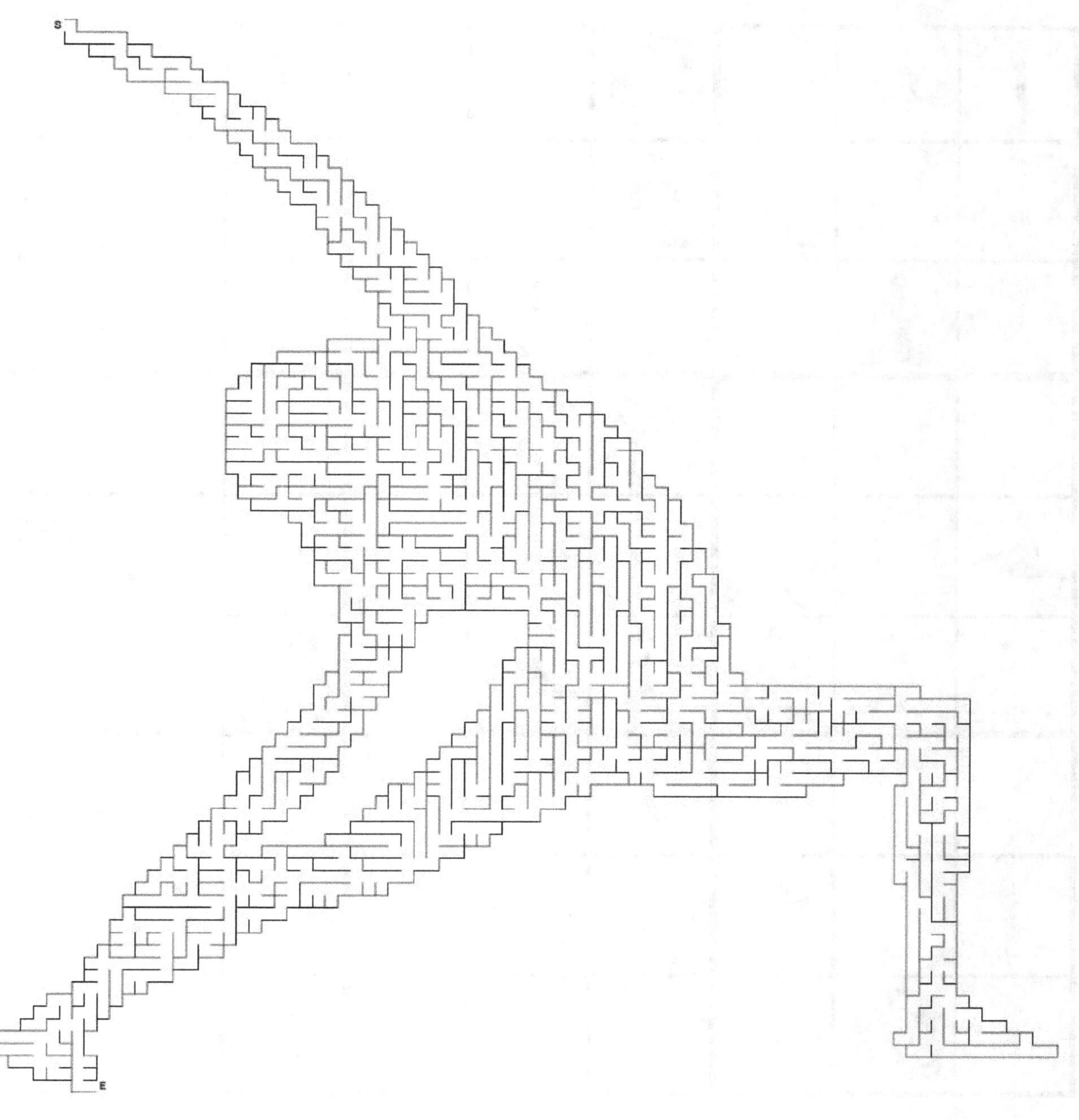

Sudoku #10

Yoga
Maze #10

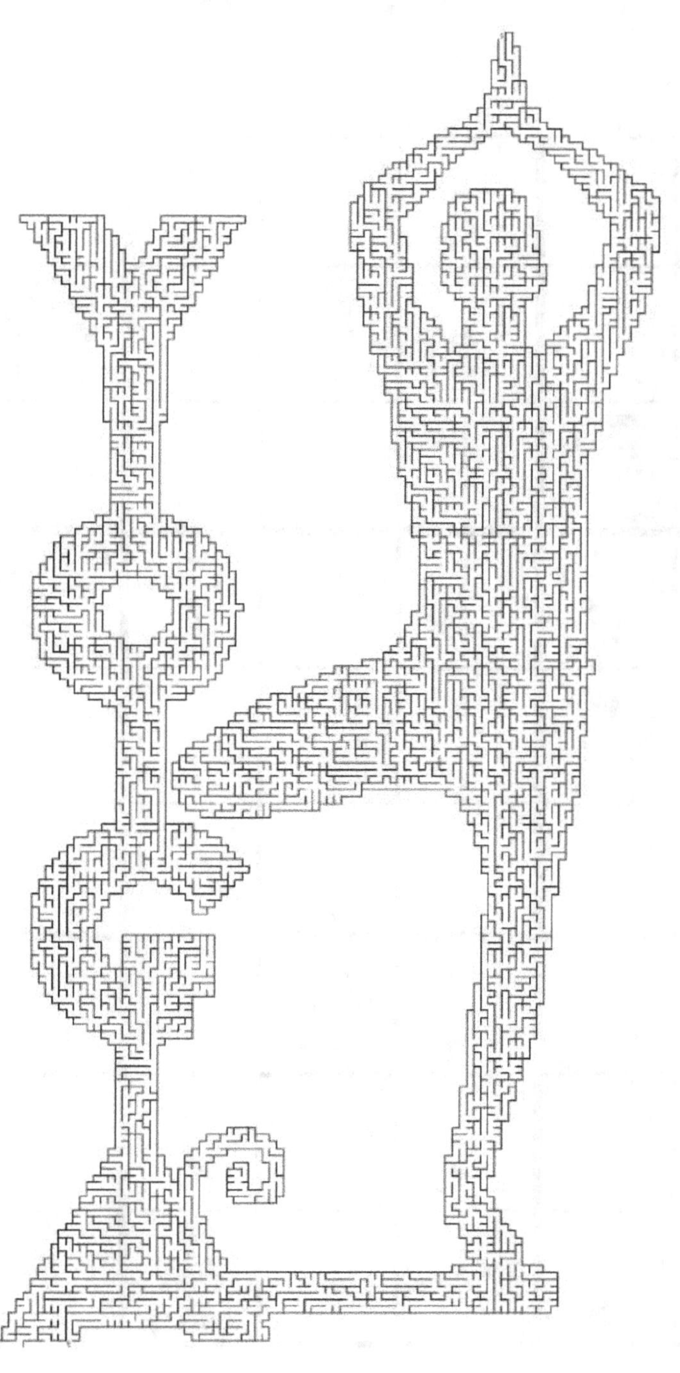

Sudoku #11

★ ★

Yoga
Maze #11

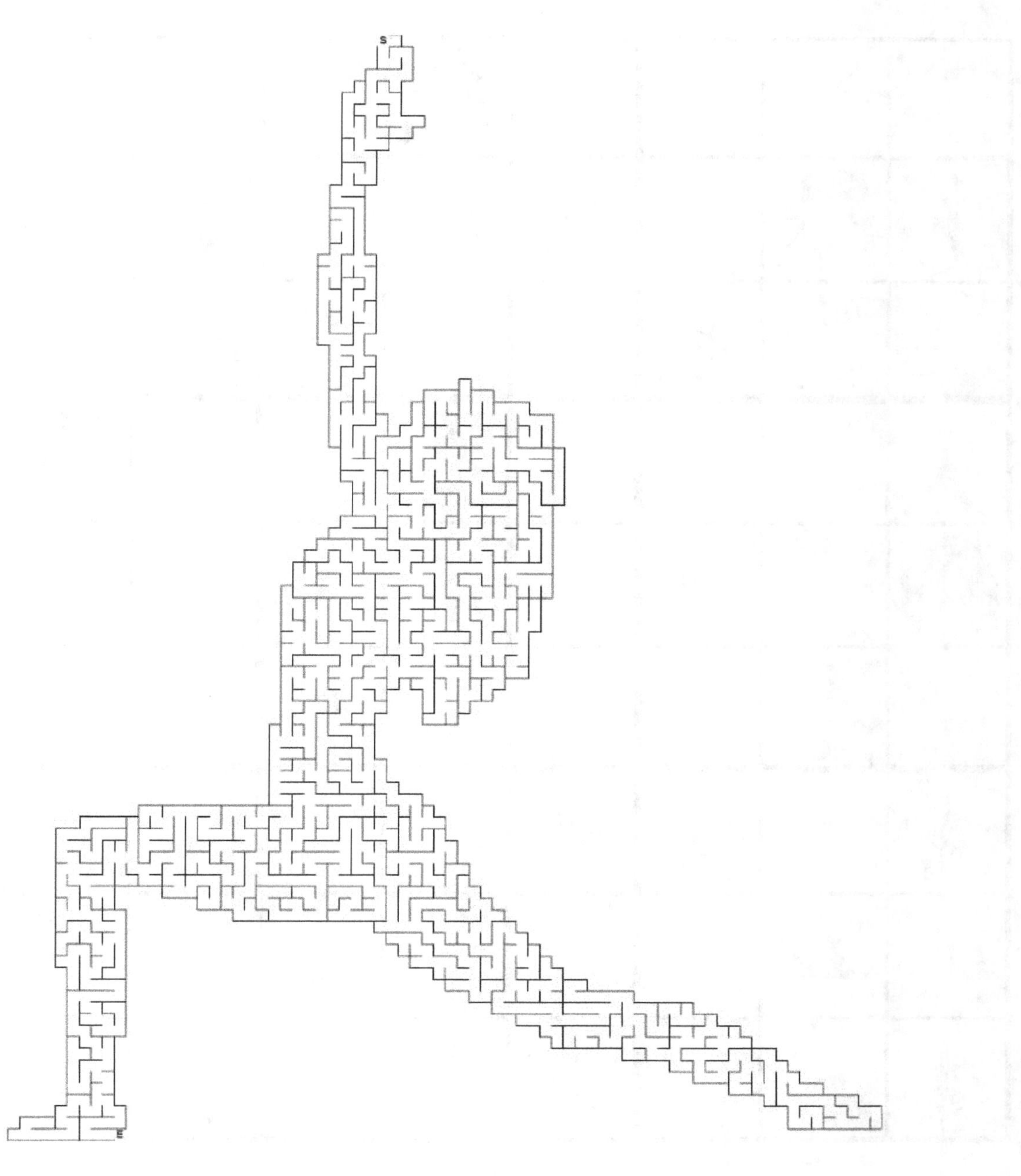

Sudoku #12

★ ★

Yoga
Maze #12

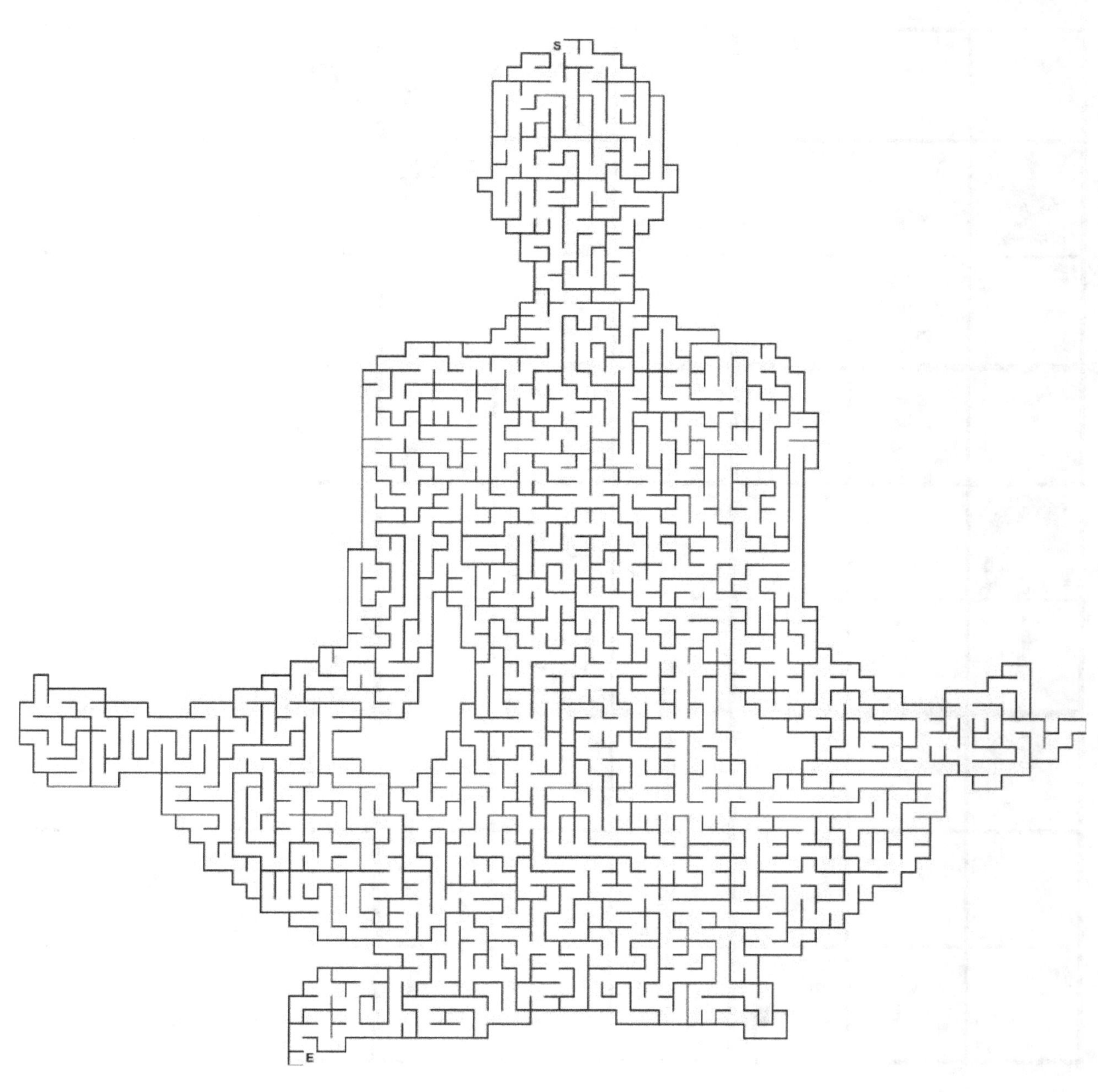

Sudoku #13

★ ★

Yoga
Maze #13

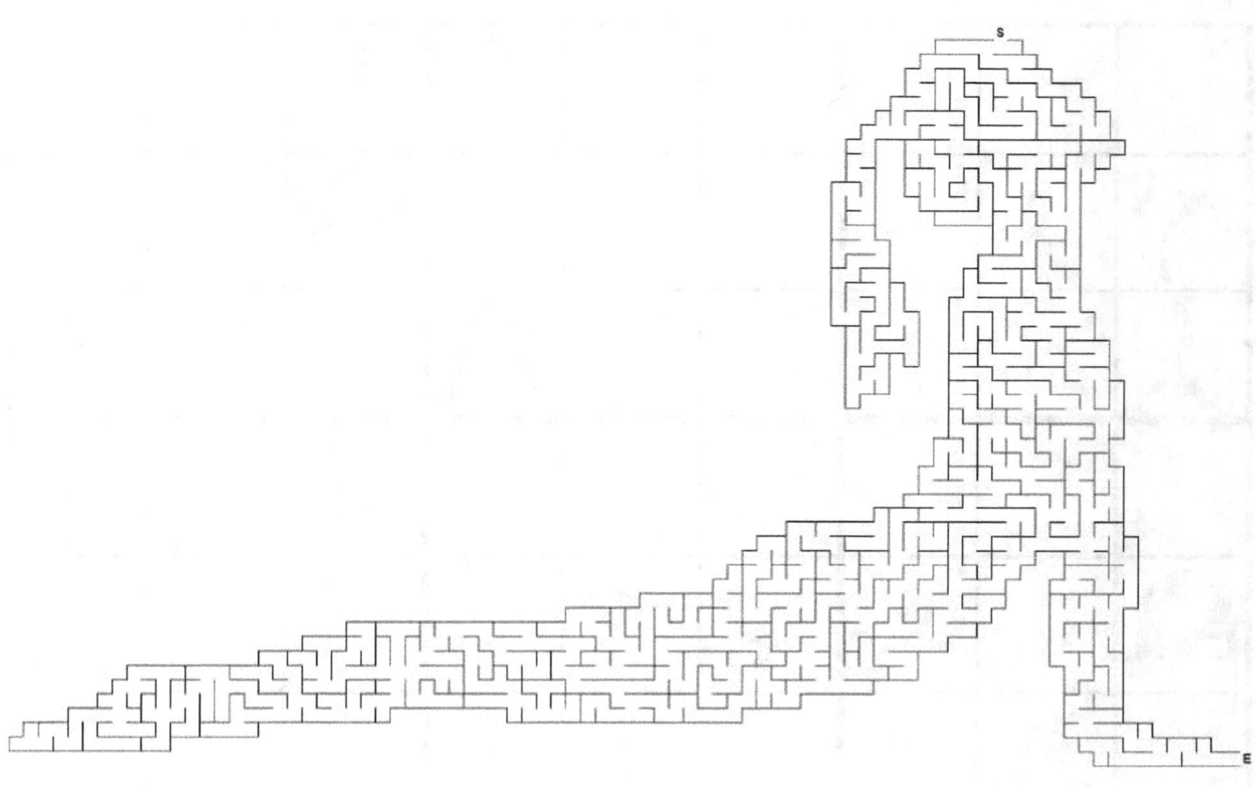

Sudoku #14

★ ★

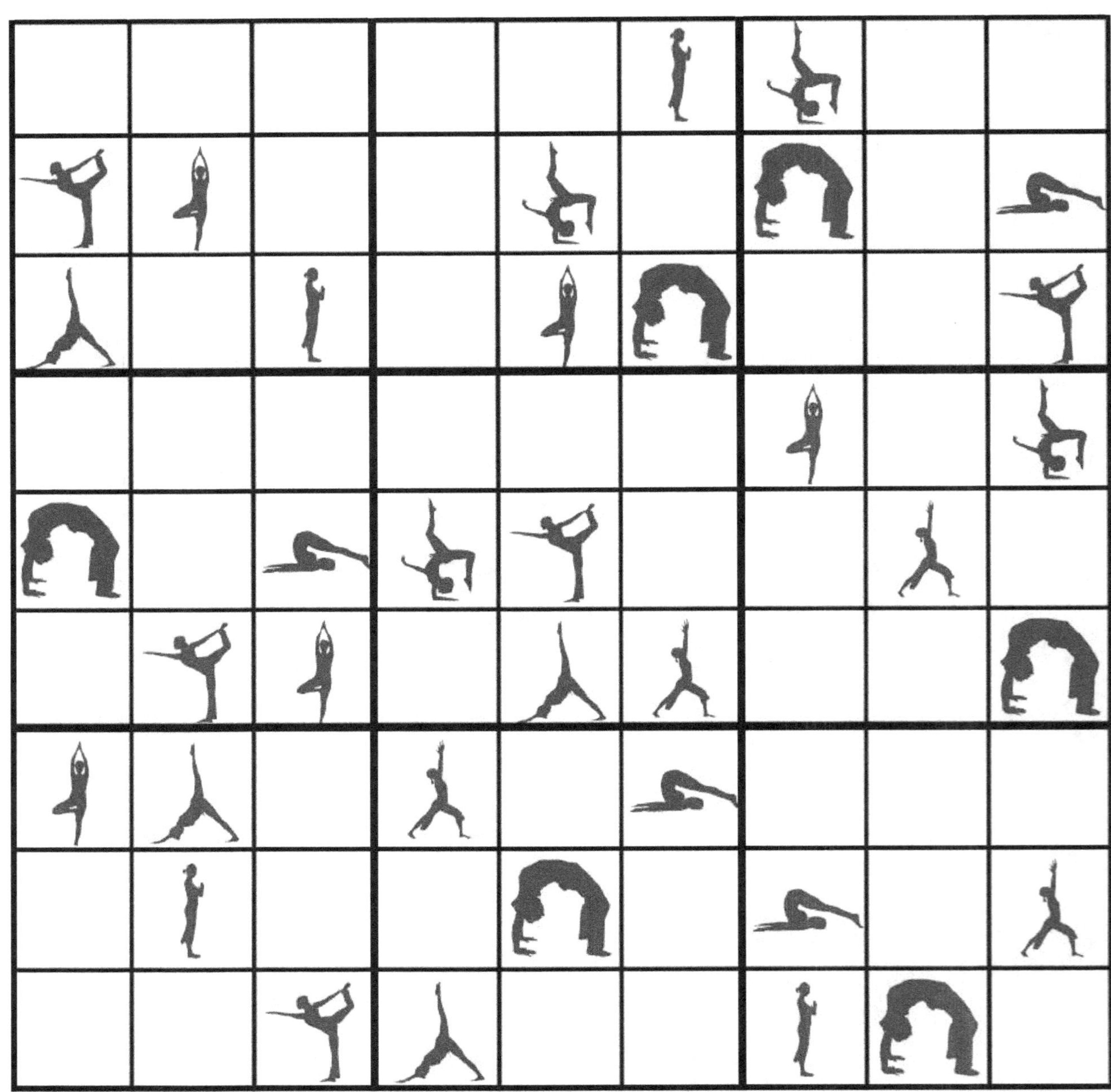

Yoga
Maze #14

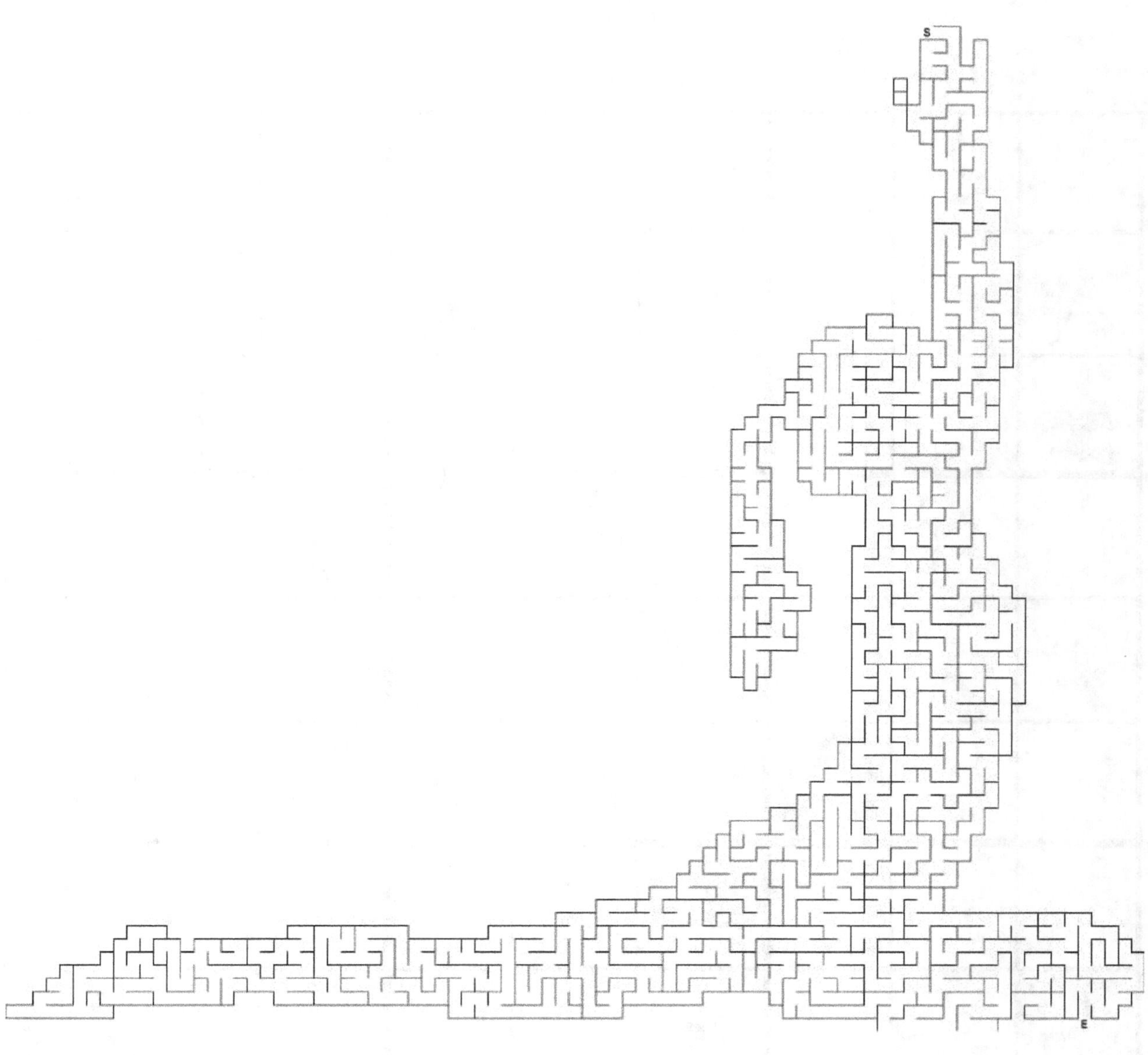

Sudoku #15

★ ★

Yoga

Maze #15

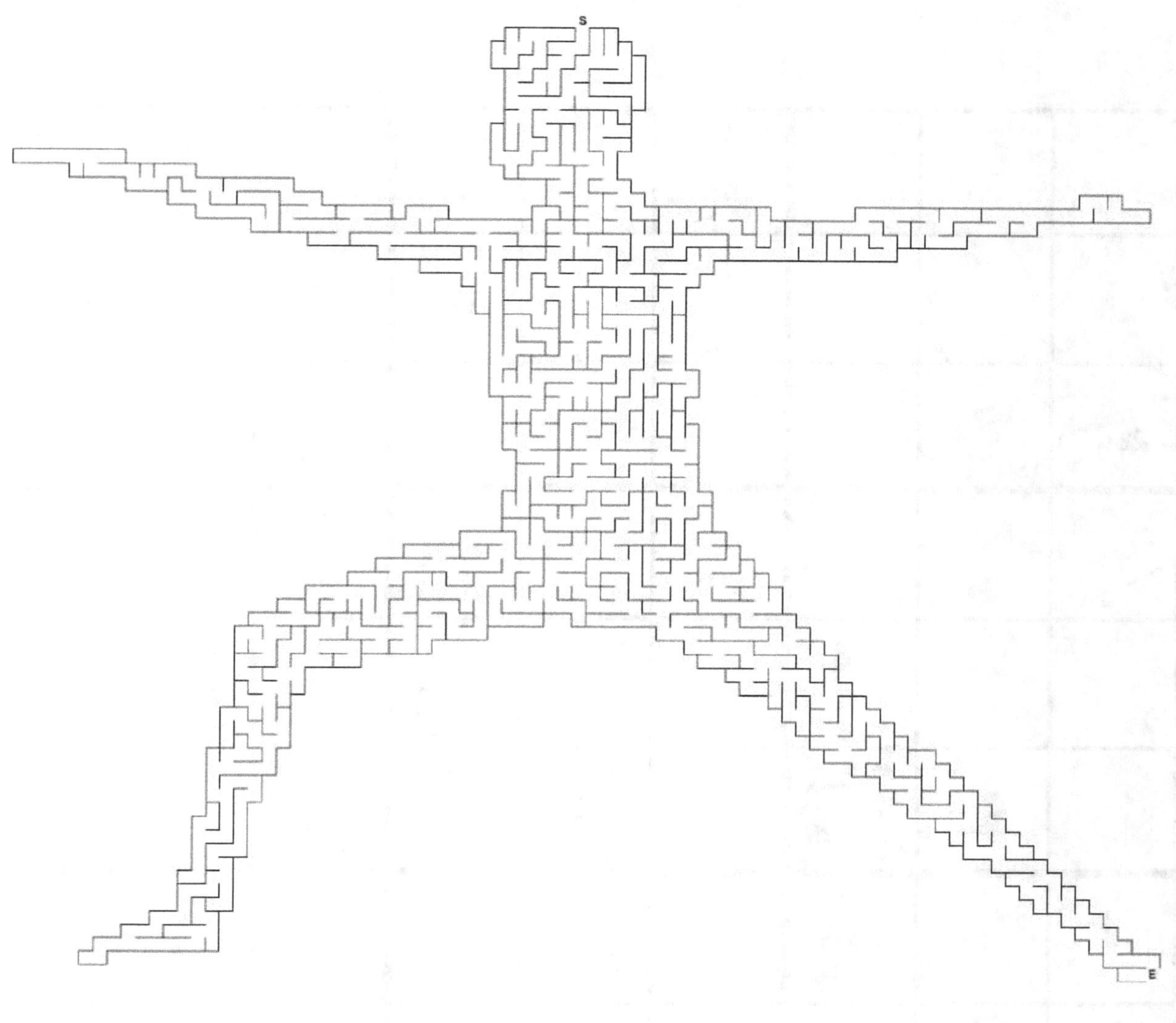

Sudoku #16

★ ★

Yoga
Maze #16

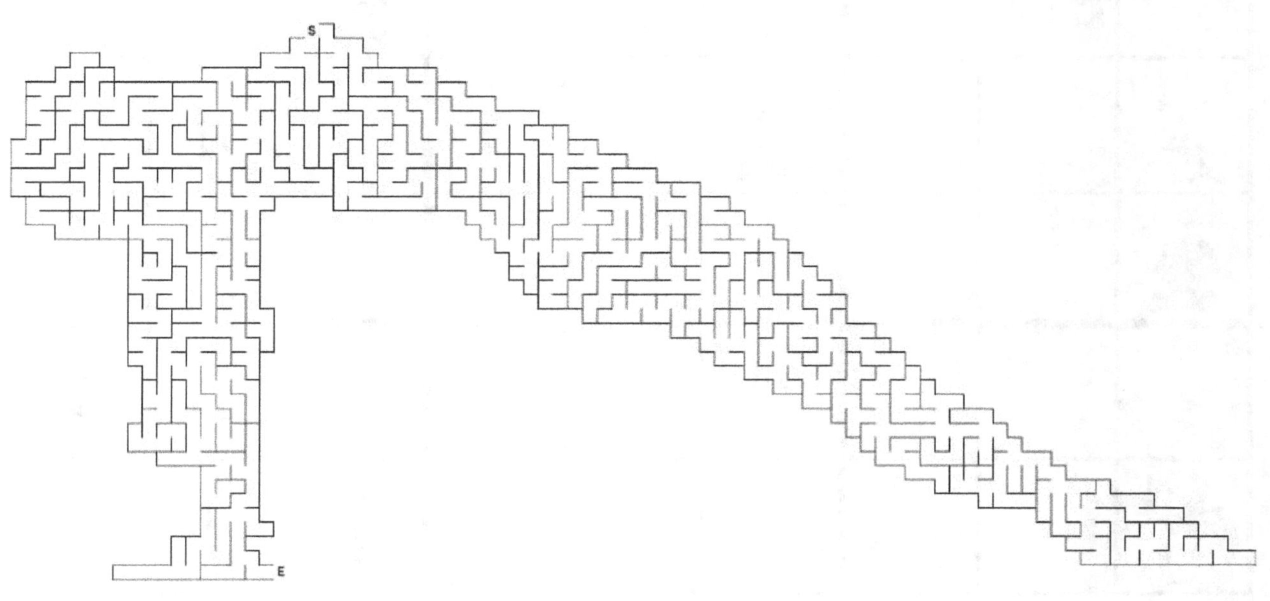

Sudoku #17

Yoga
Maze #17

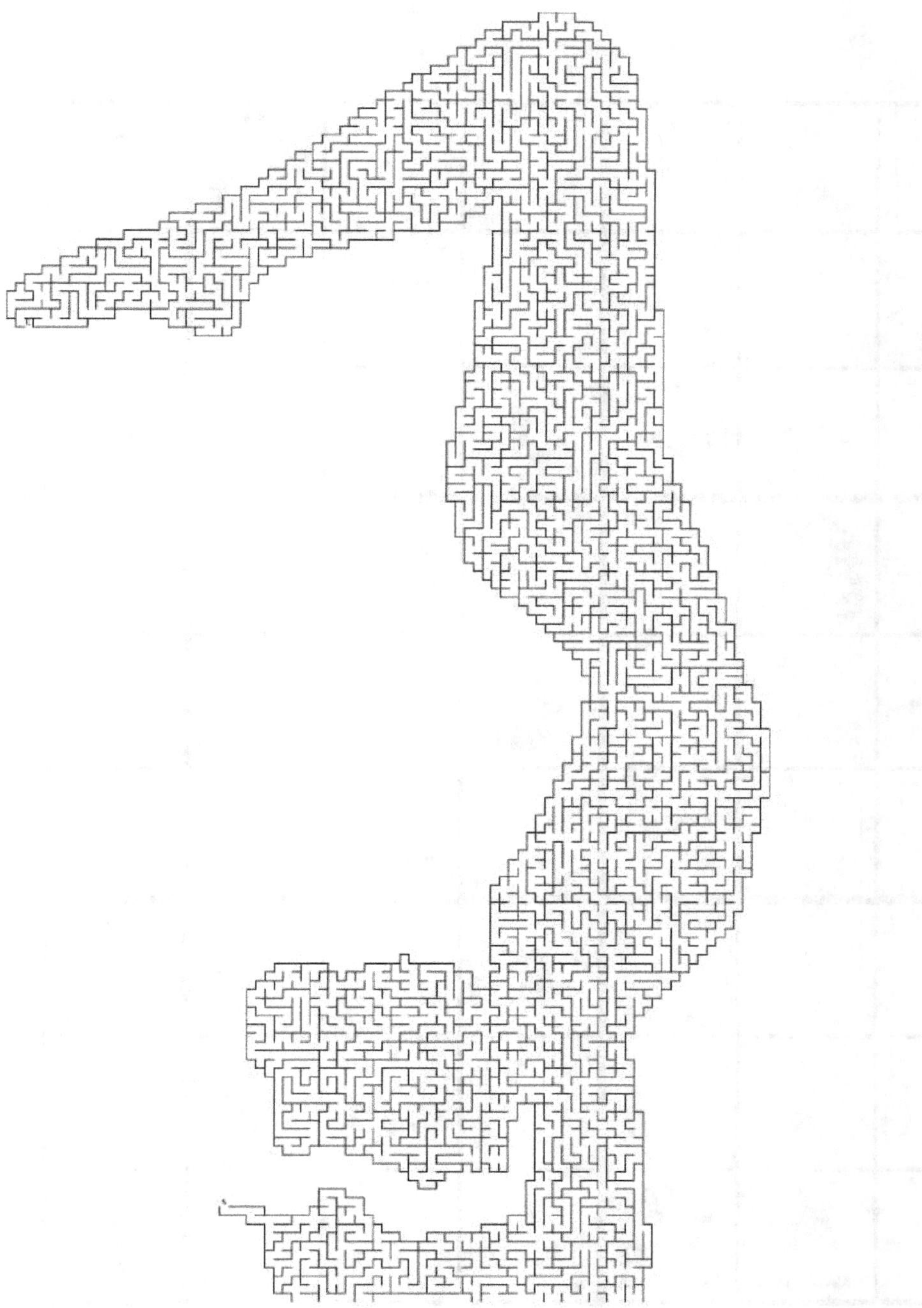

Sudoku #18

★★

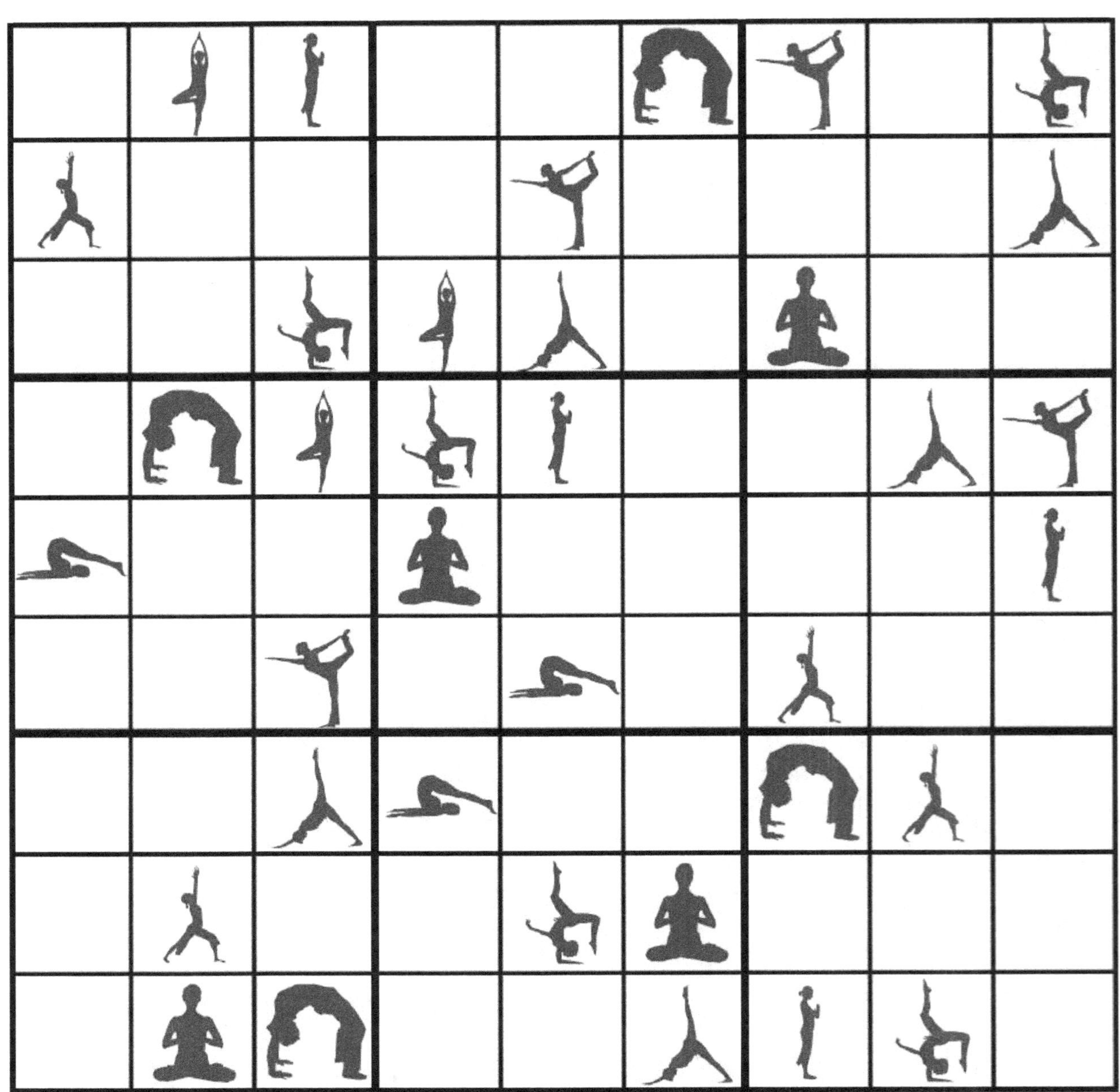

Yoga

Maze #18

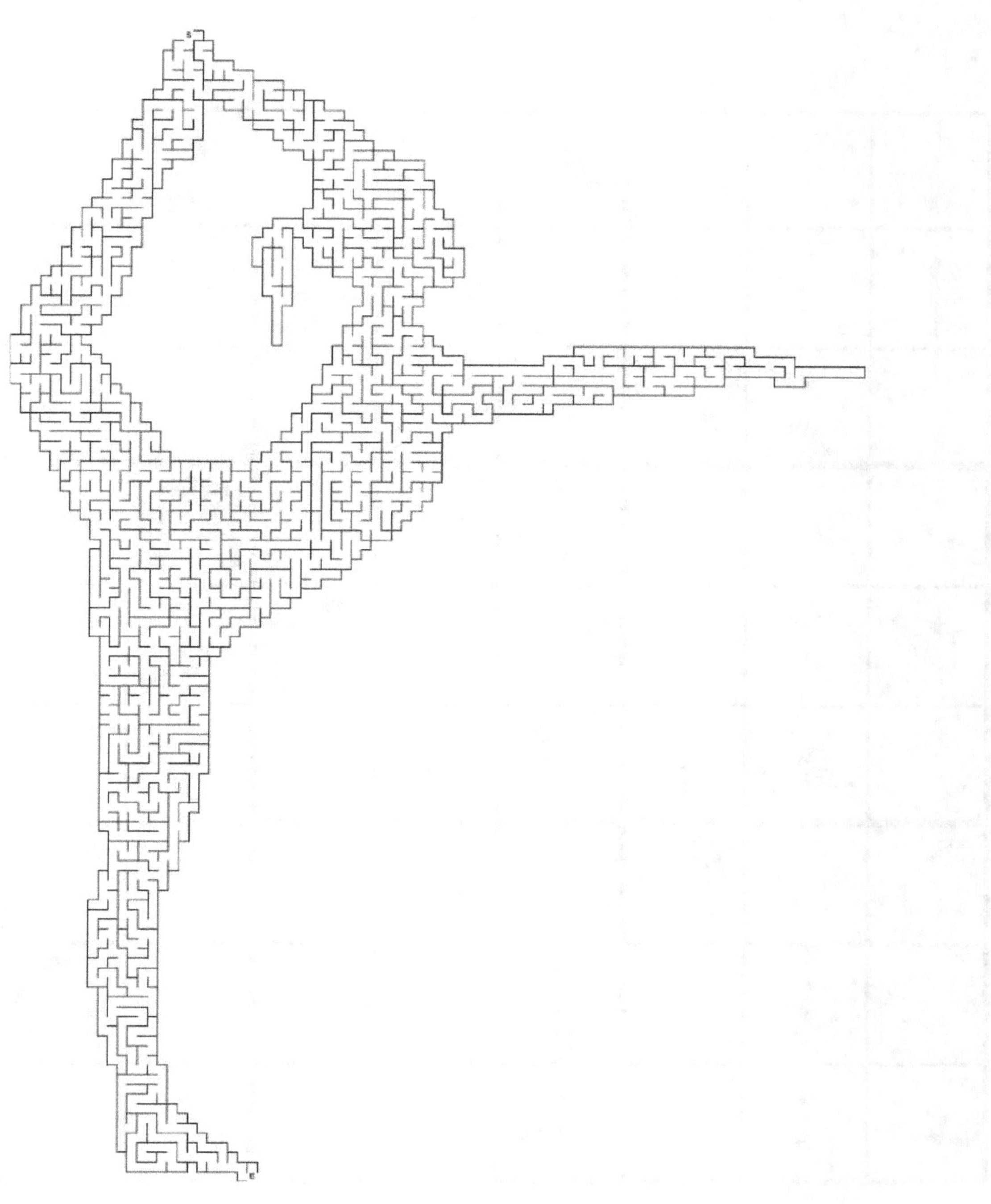

Sudoku #19

★ ★

Yoga

Maze #19

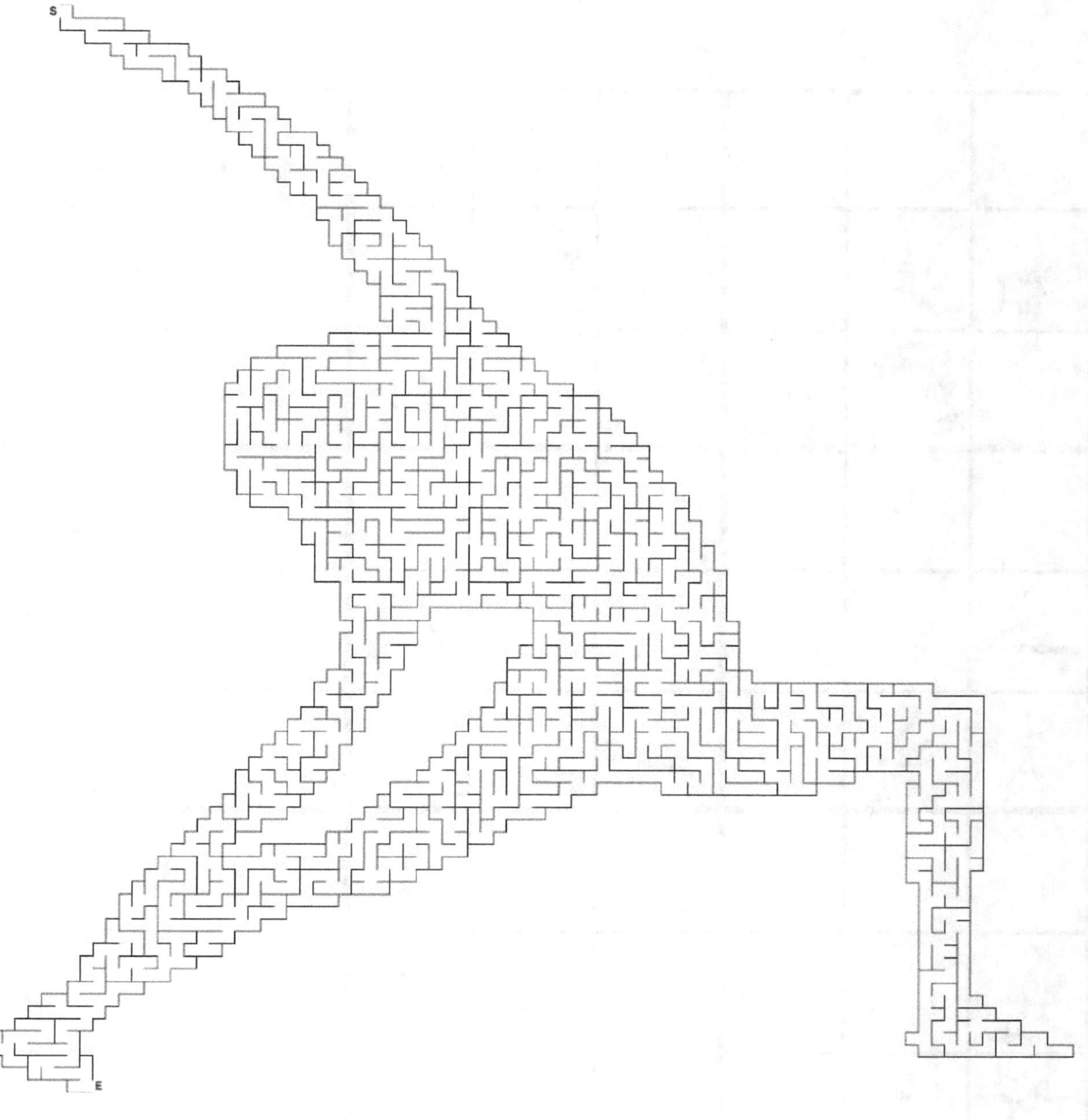

Sudoku #20

★ ★

Yoga
Maze #20

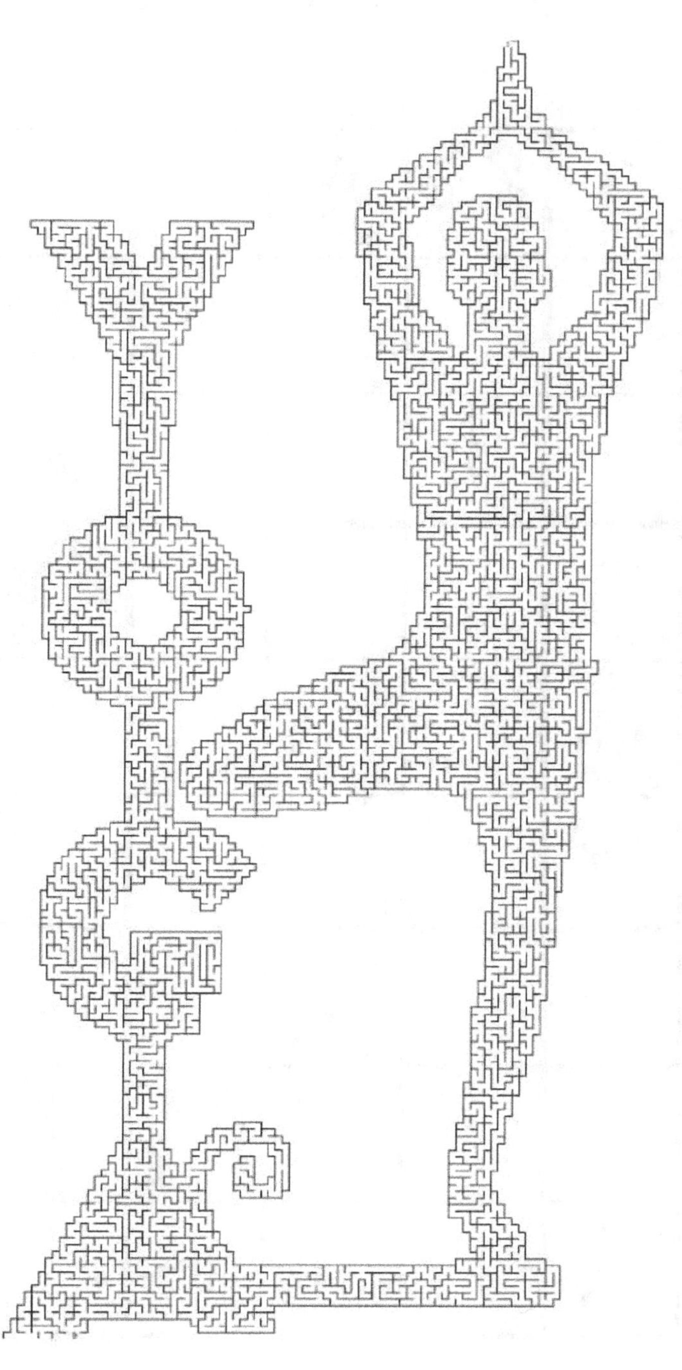

Sudoku #21

★★★

Yoga
Maze #21

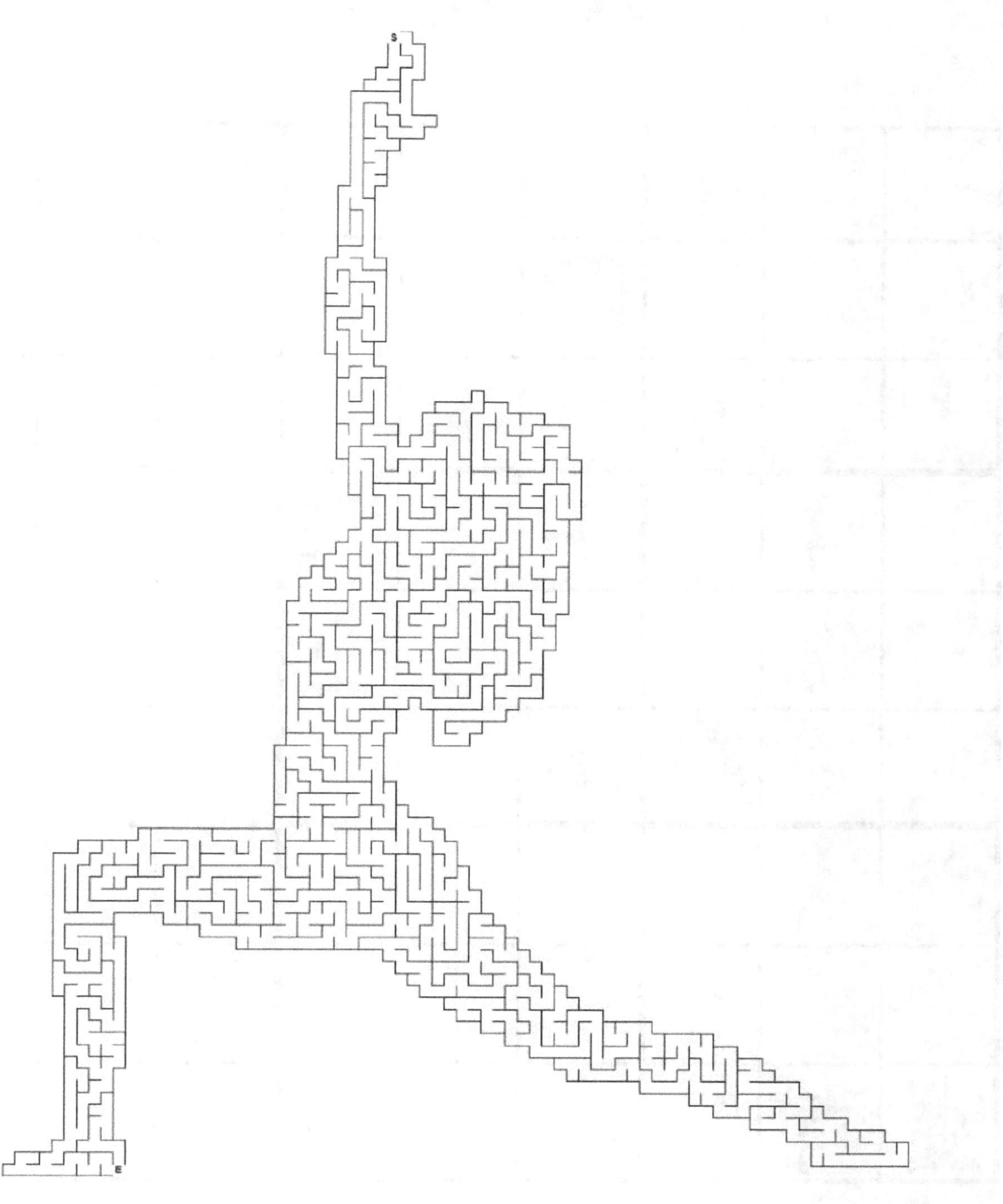

Sudoku #22

Yoga

Maze #22

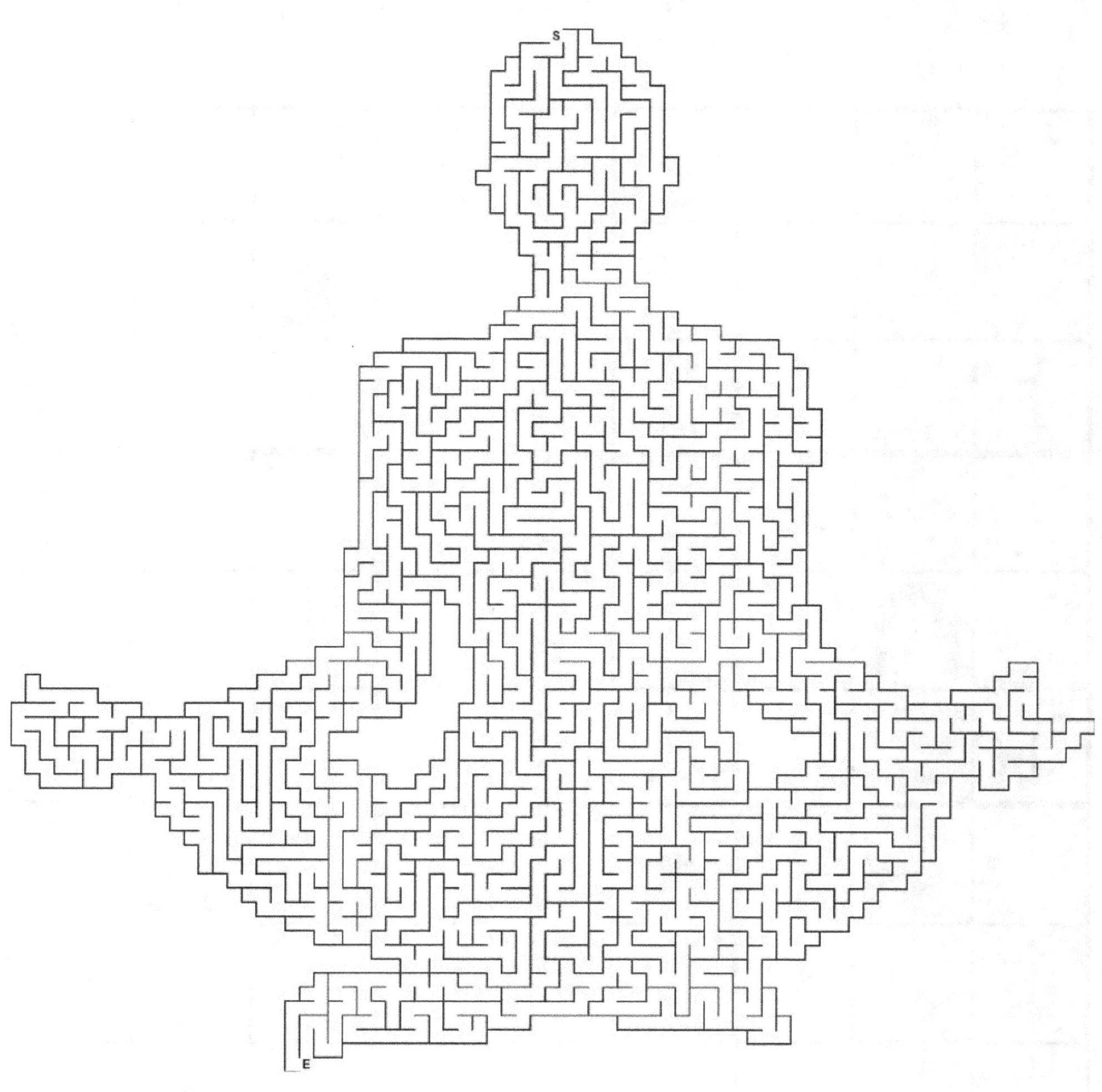

Sudoku #23

★★★

Yoga
Maze #23

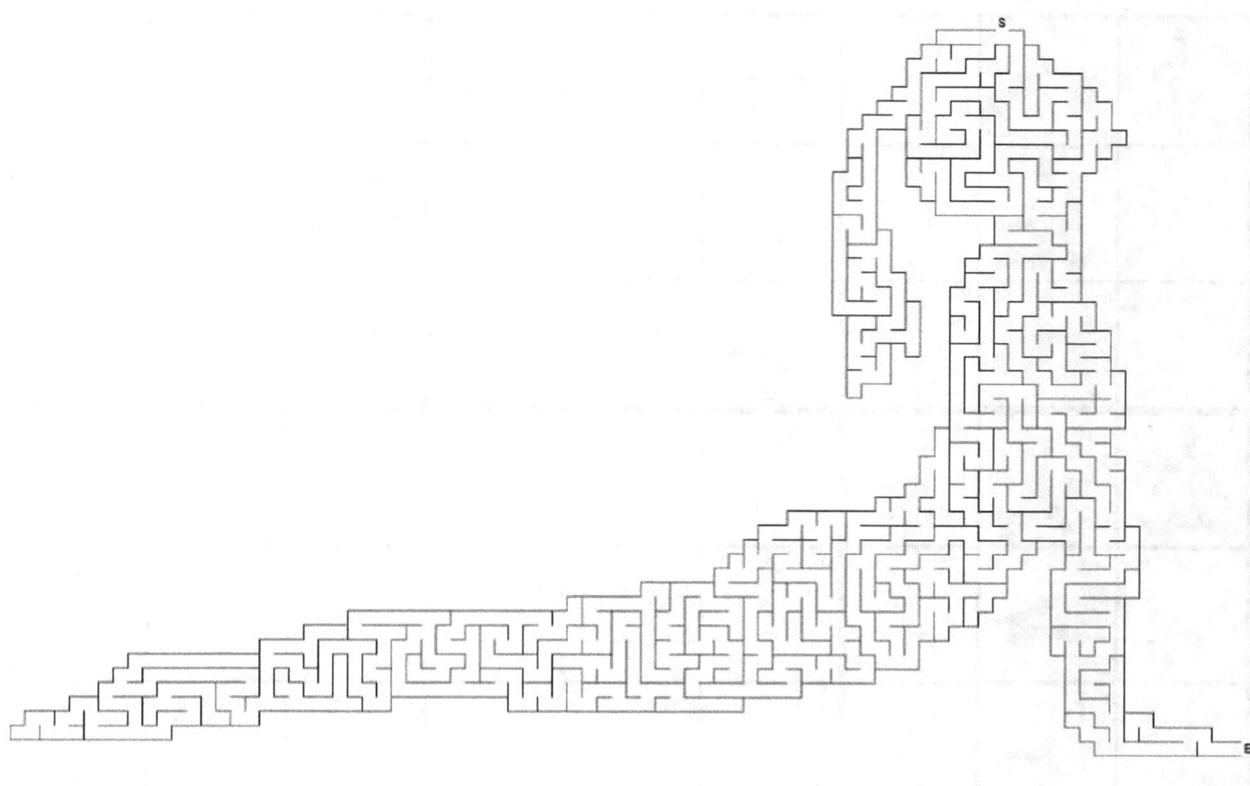

Sudoku #24

★★★

Yoga

Maze #24

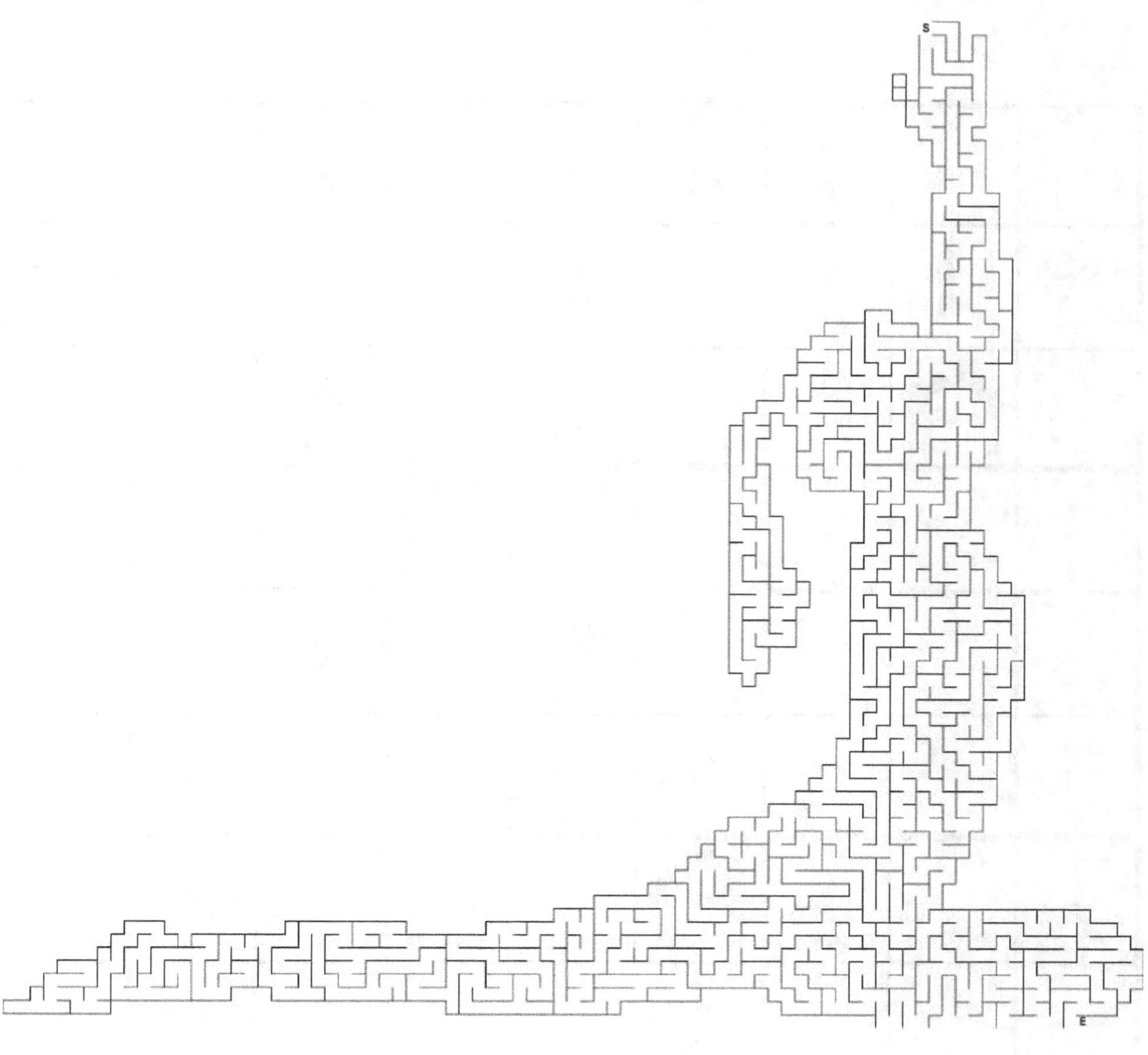

Sudoku #25

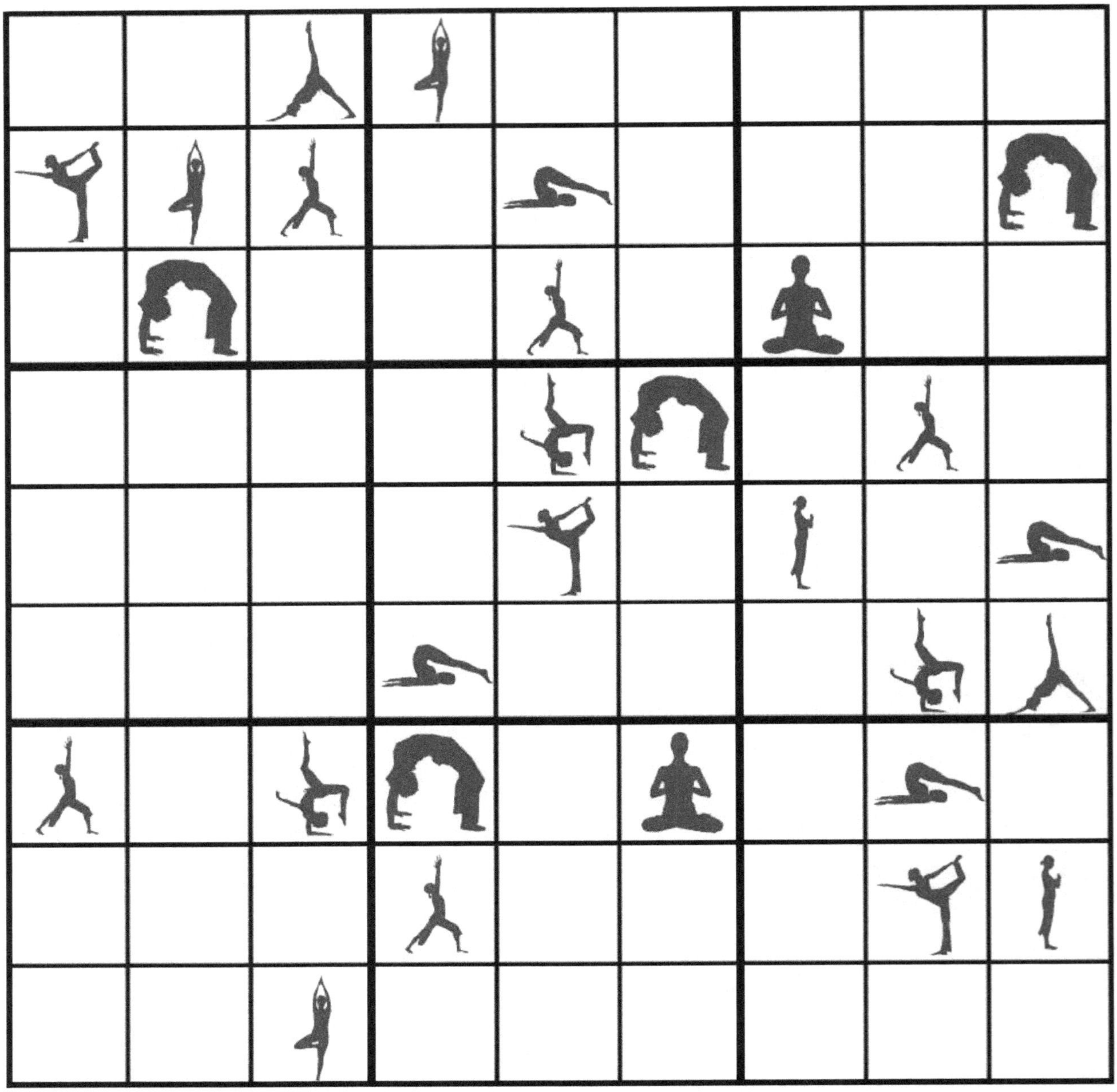

★★★

Yoga
Maze #25

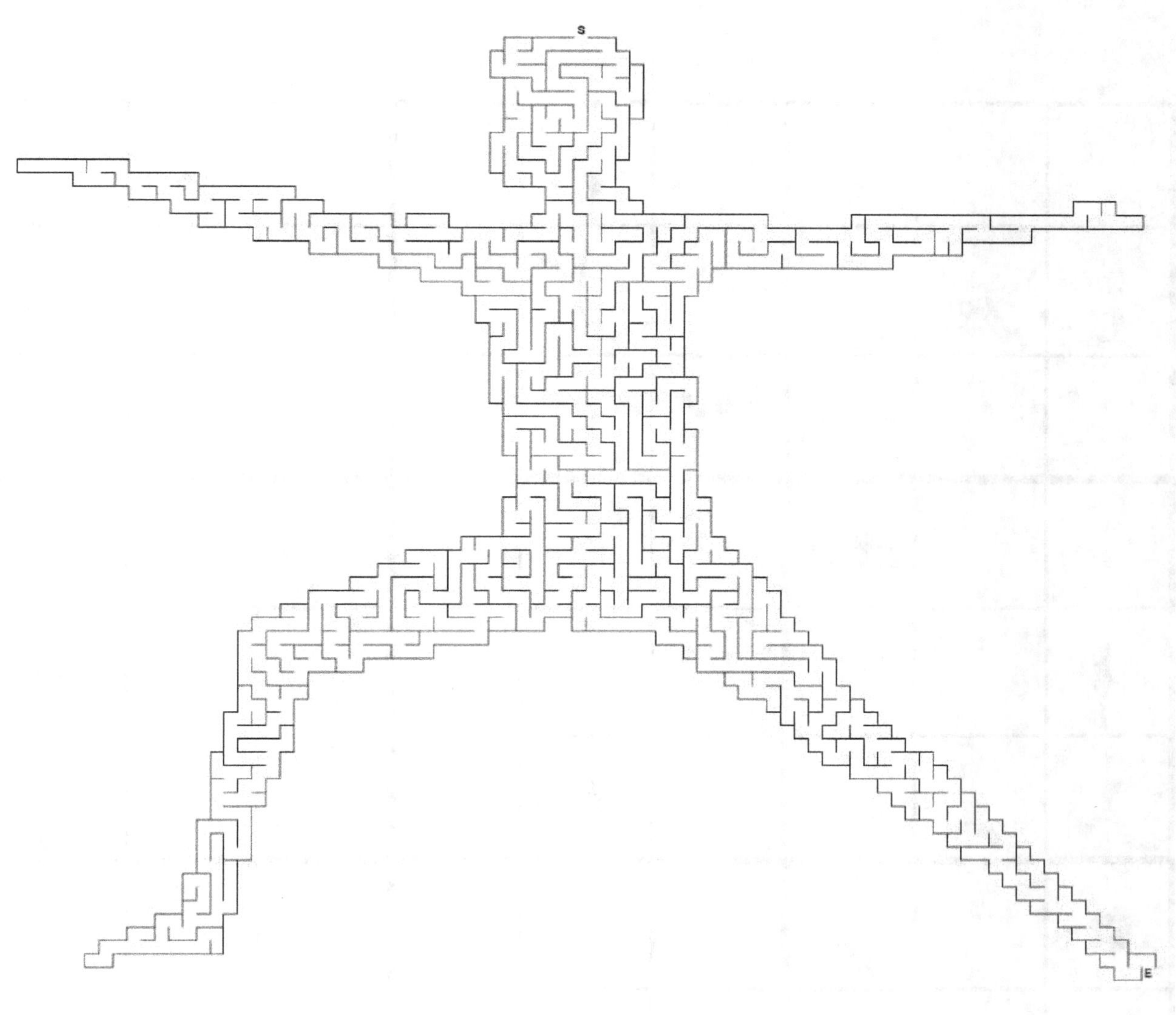

Sudoku #26

★★★

Yoga

Maze #26

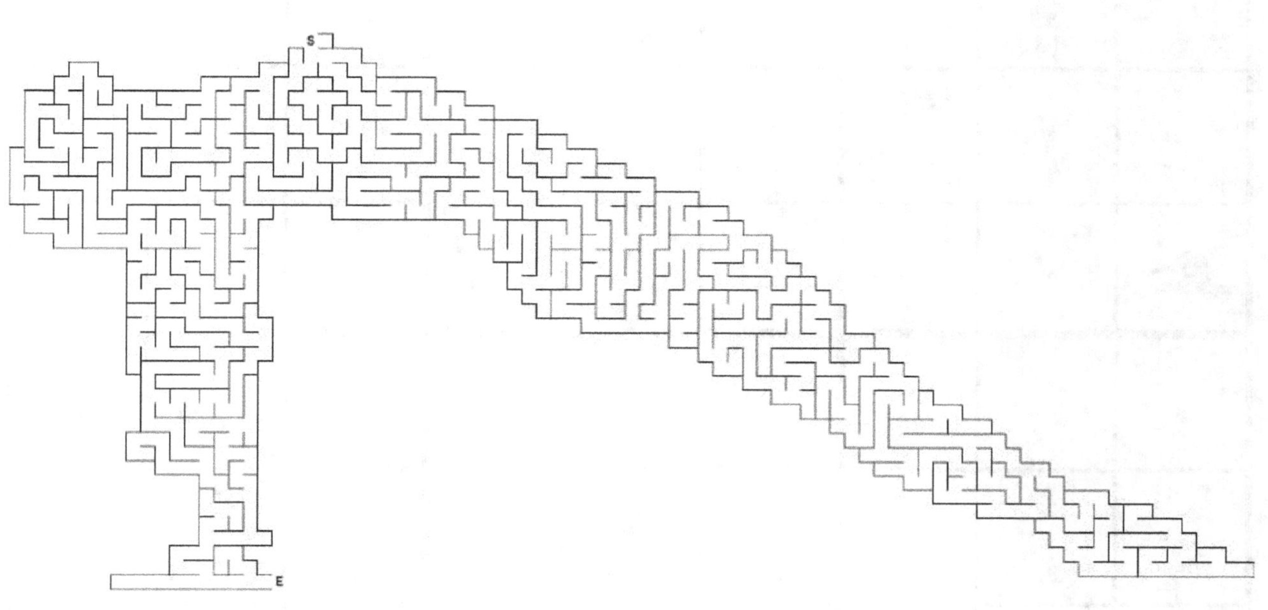

Sudoku #27

★★★

Yoga
Maze #27

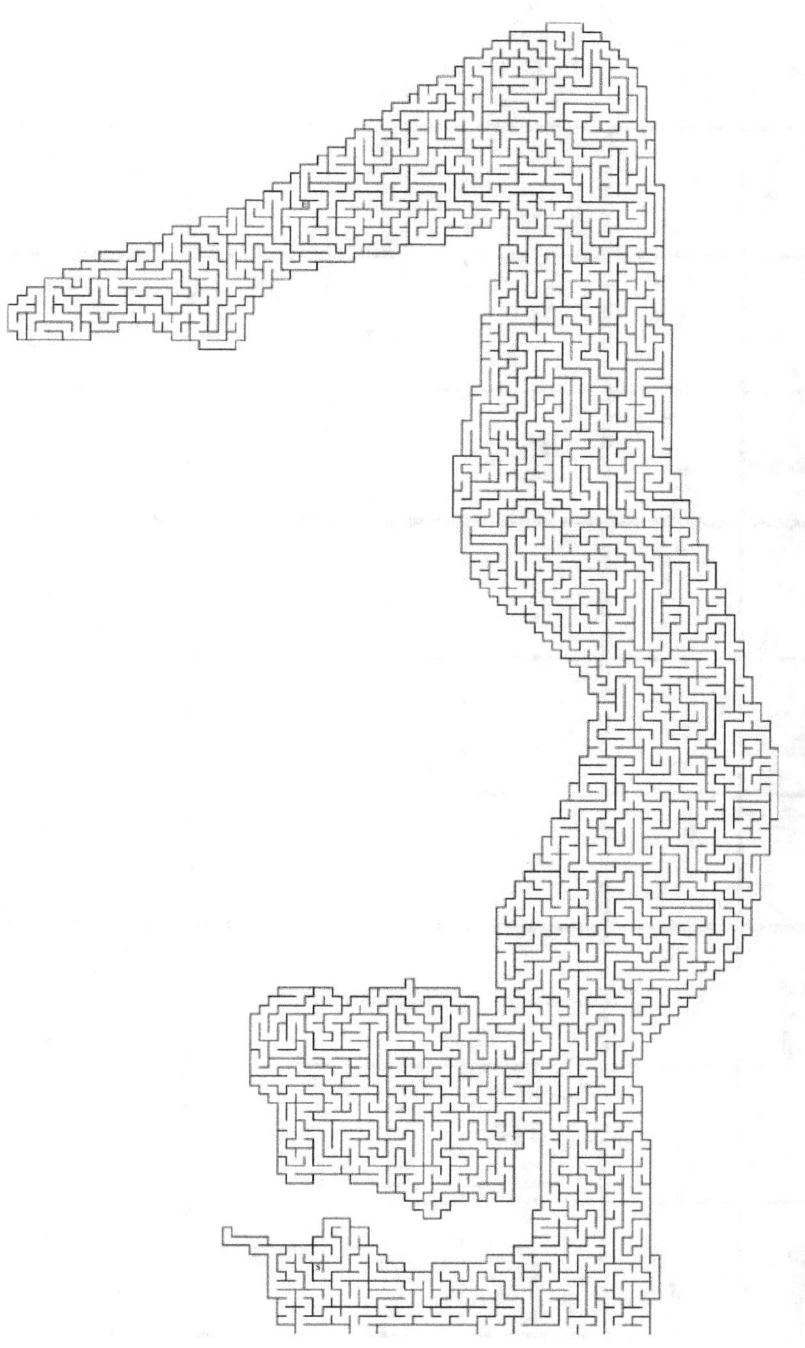

Sudoku #28

★★★

Yoga
Maze #28

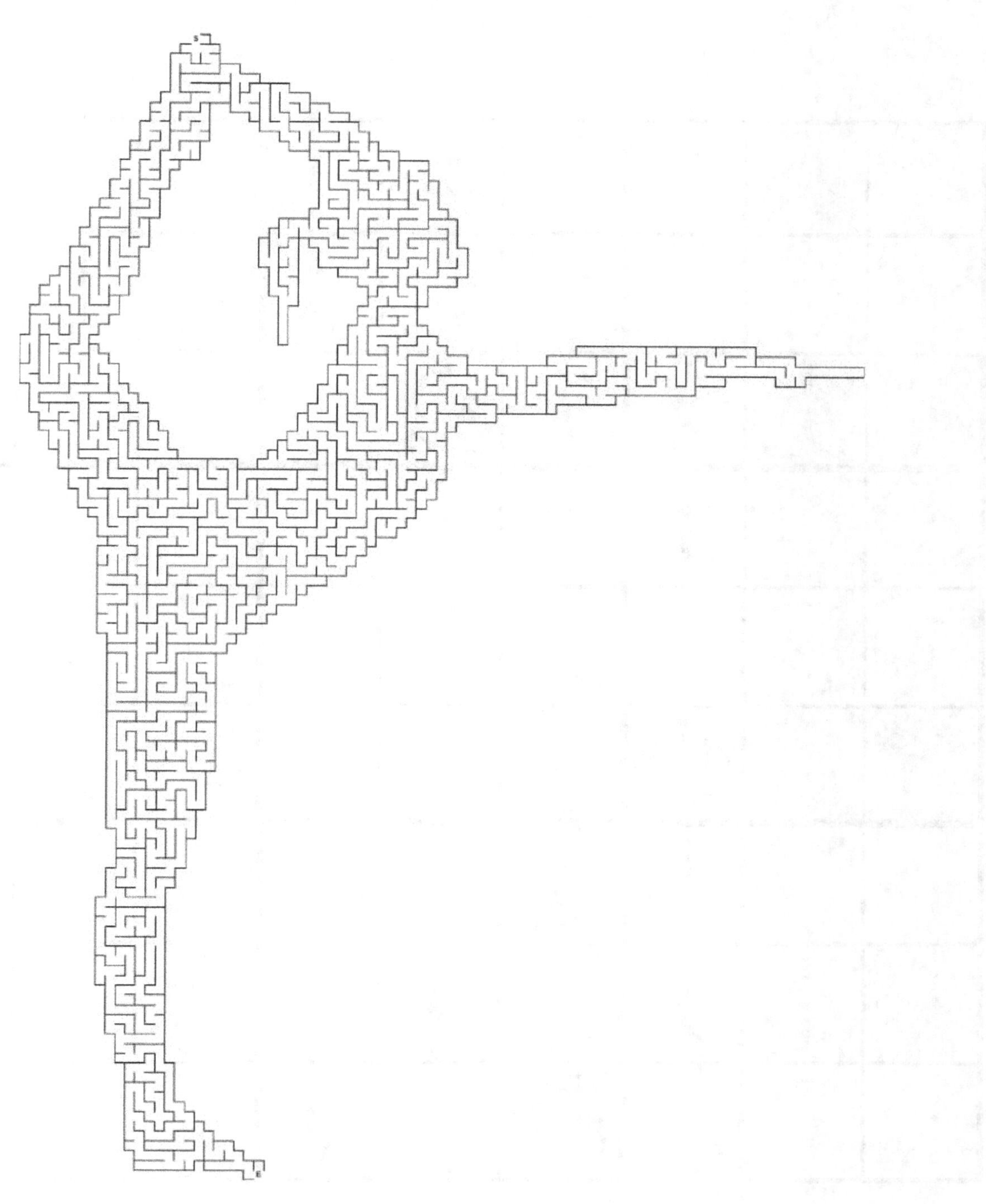

Sudoku #29

Yoga
Maze #29

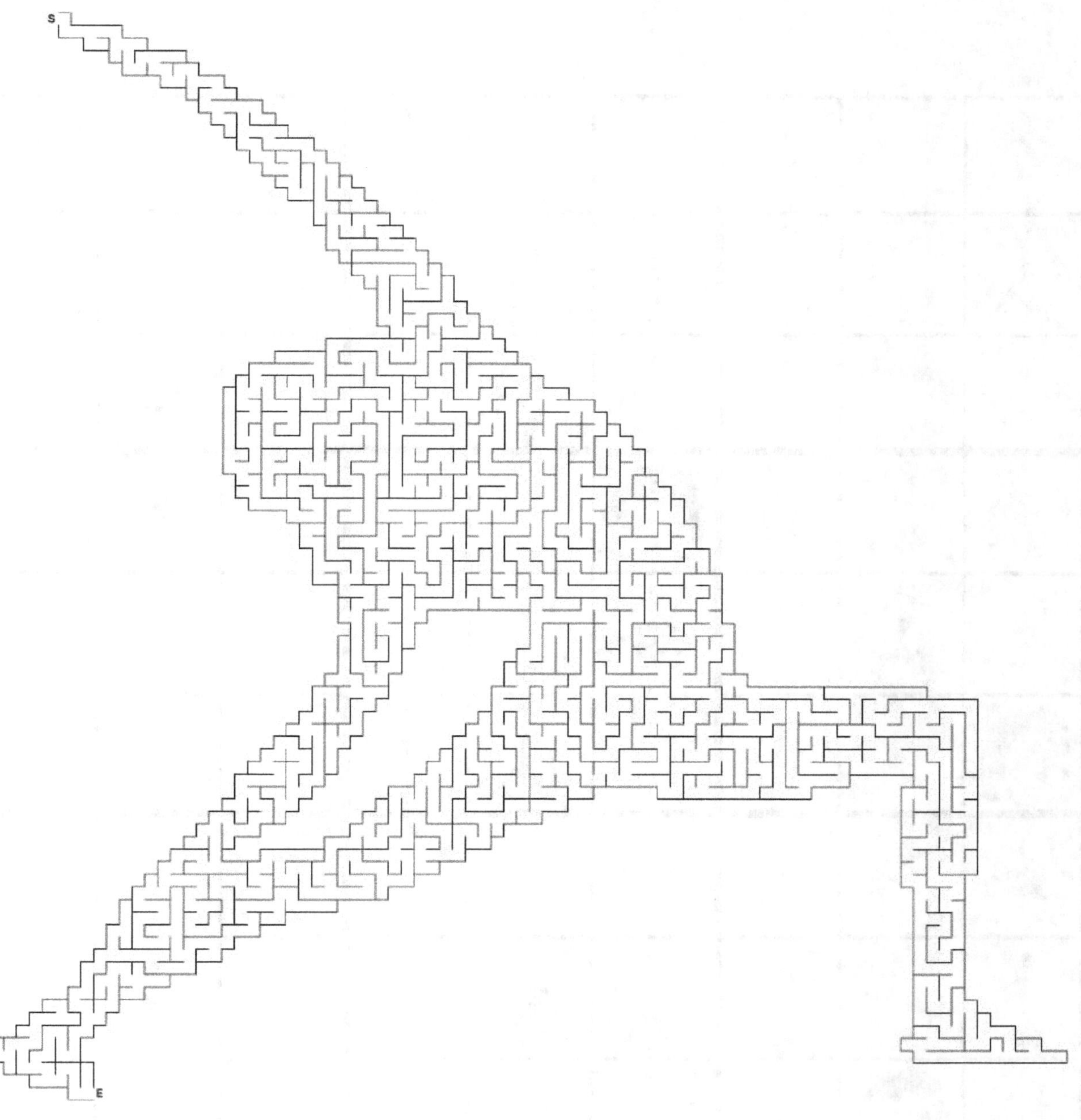

Sudoku #30

★ ★ ★

Yoga
Maze #30

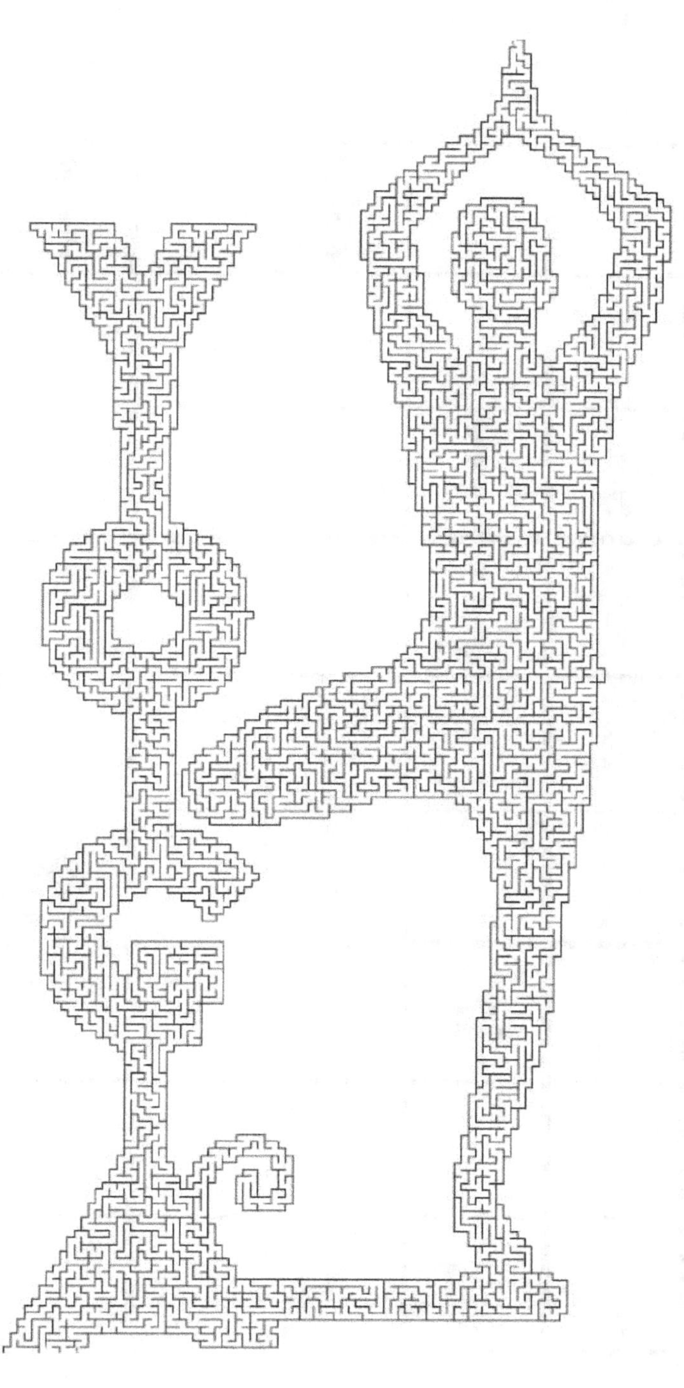

Sudoku #31

★★★★

Yoga
Maze #31

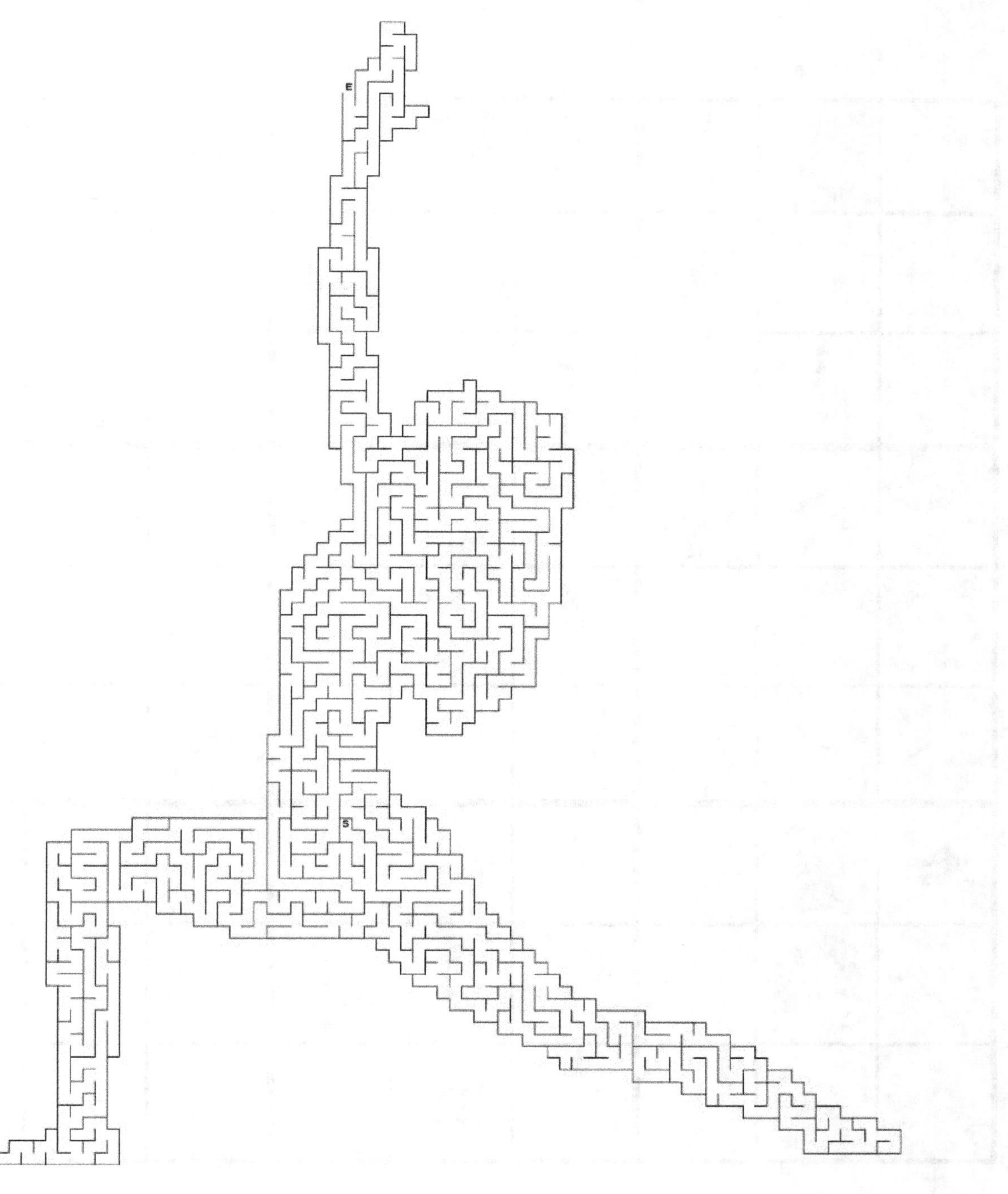

Sudoku #32

★★★★

Yoga
Maze #32

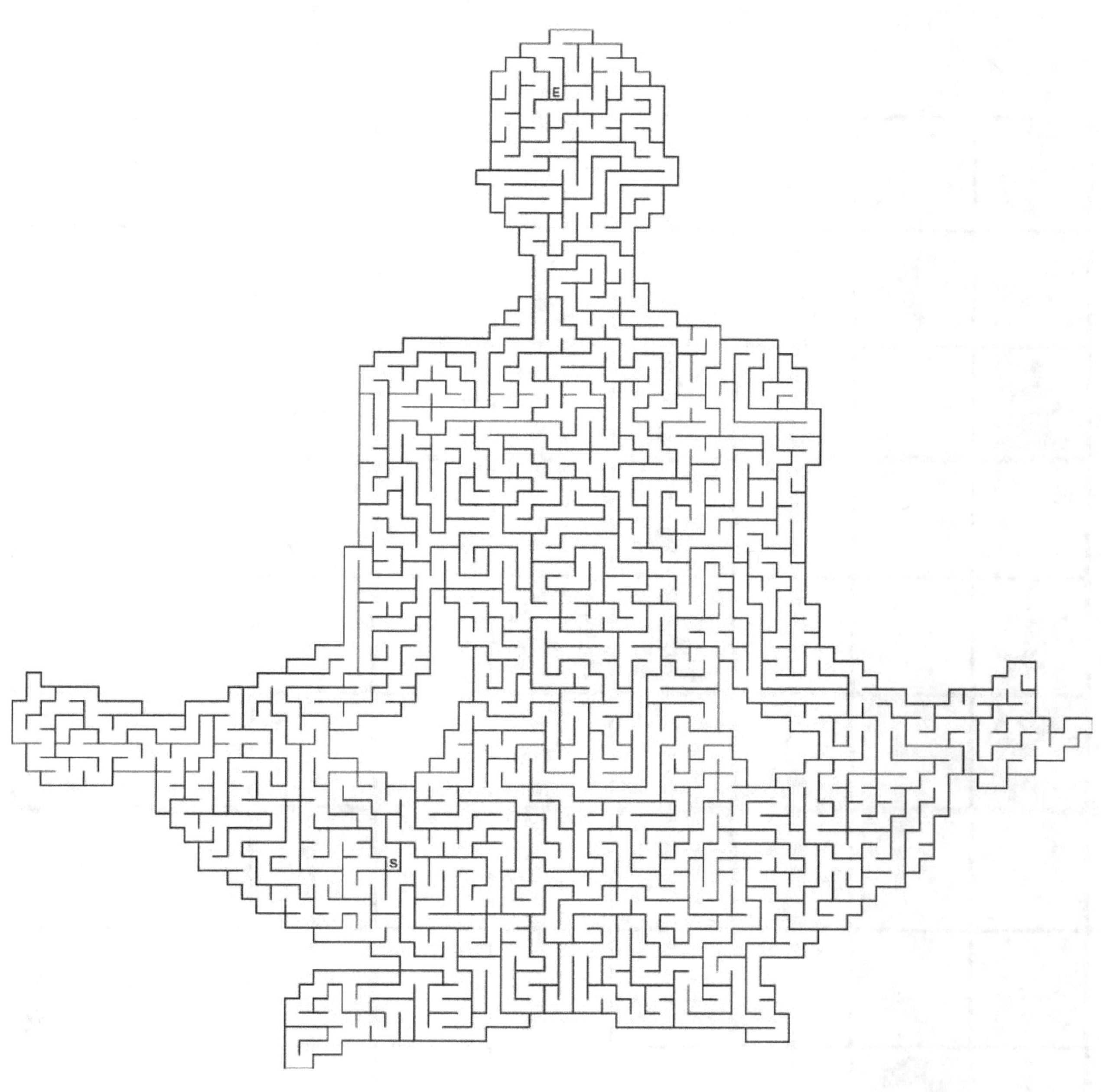

Sudoku #33

★★★★★

Yoga
Maze #33

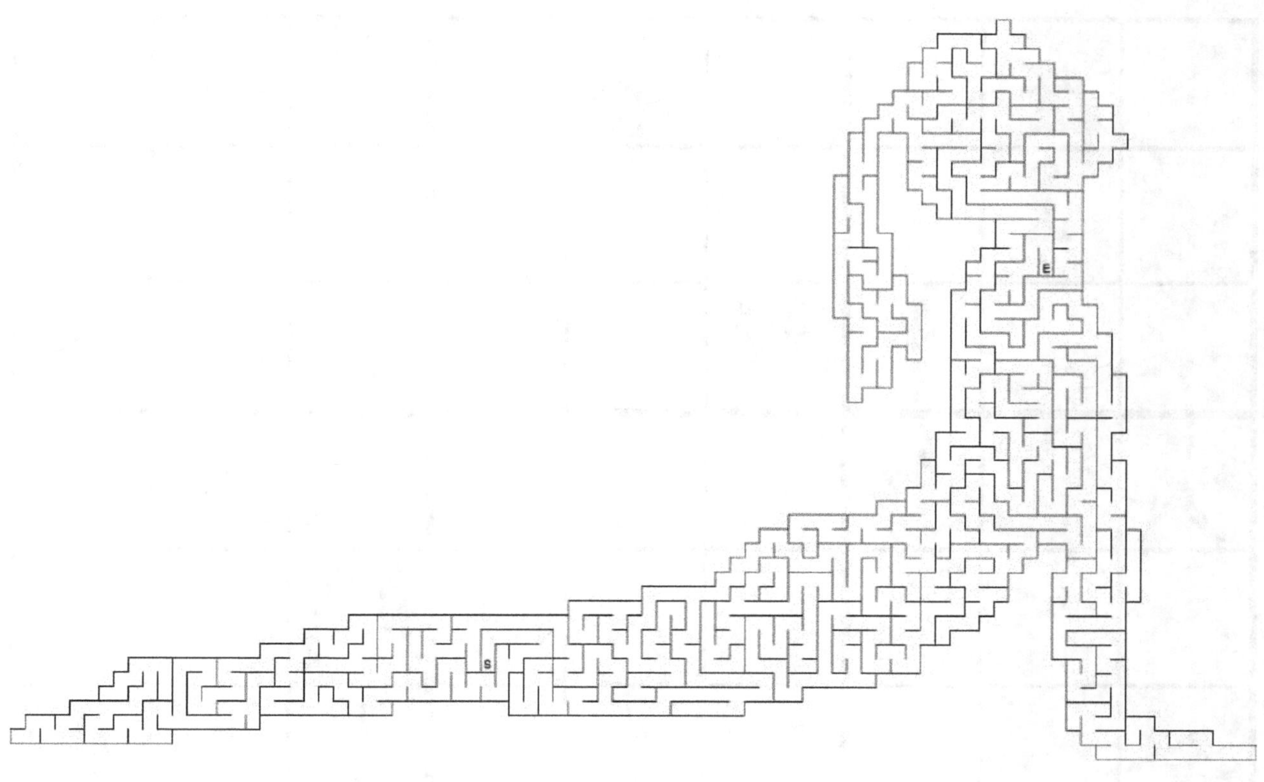

Sudoku #34

★★★★

Yoga
Maze #34

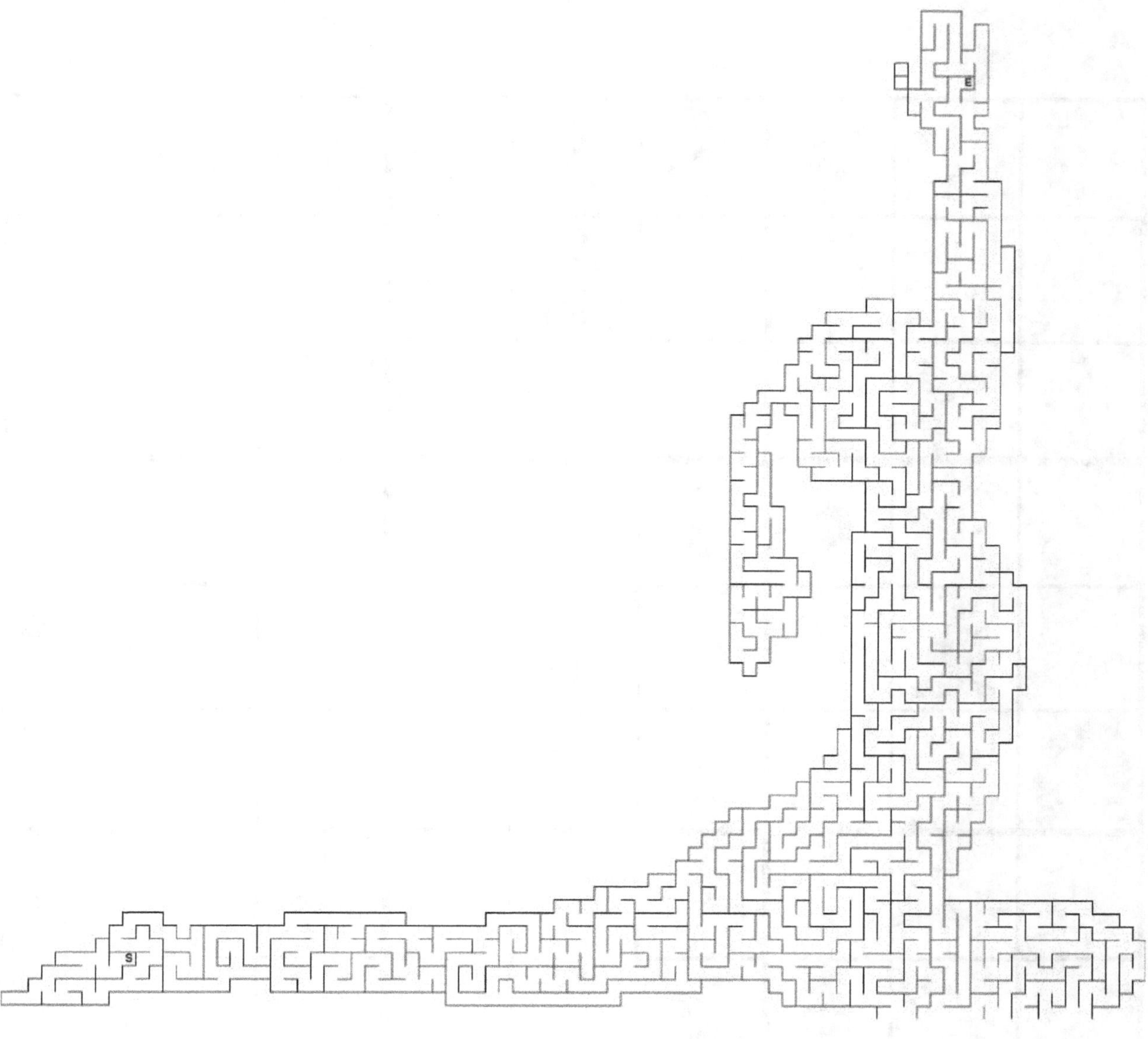

Sudoku #35

★★★★★

Yoga
Maze #35

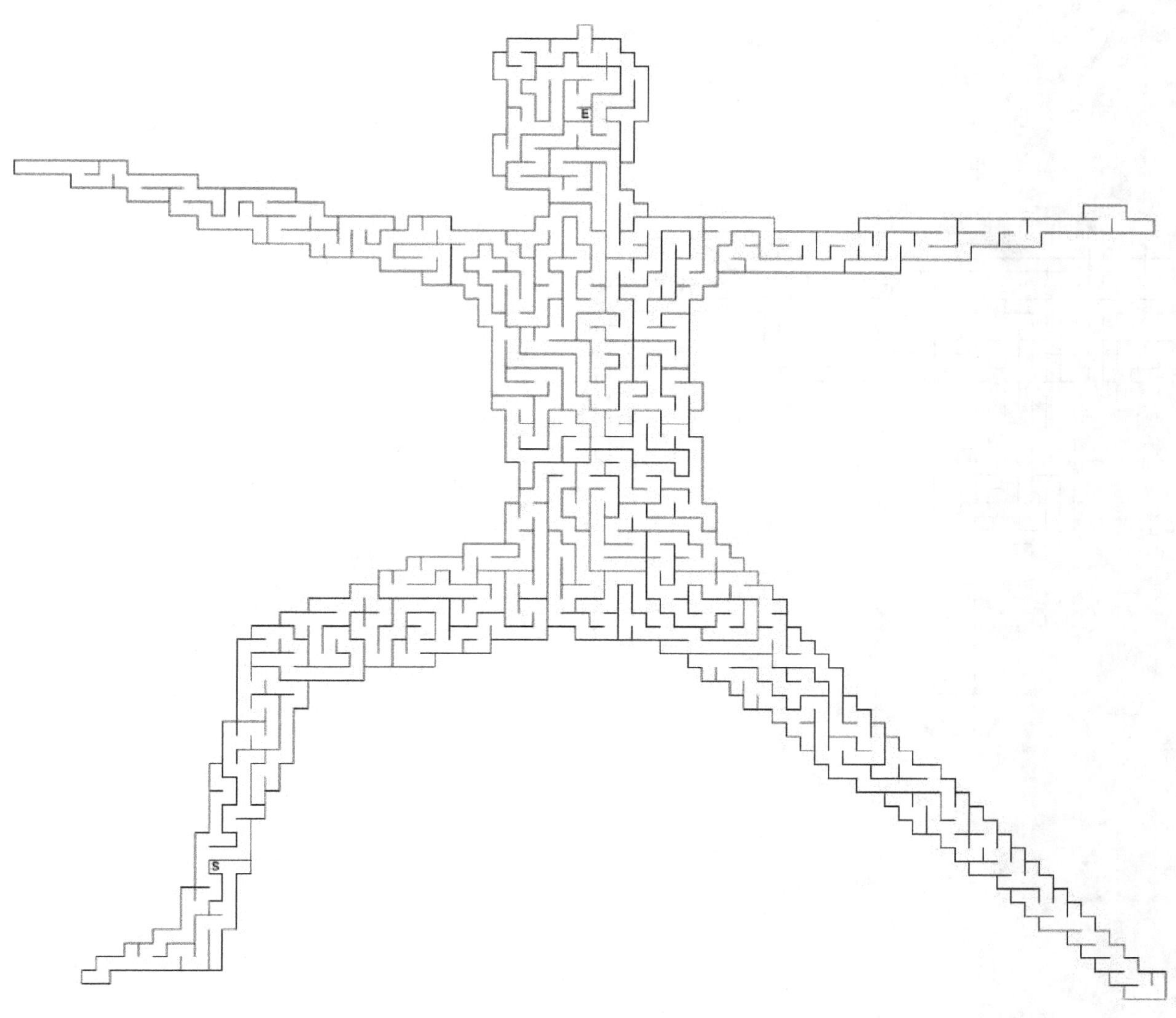

Yoga
Maze #36

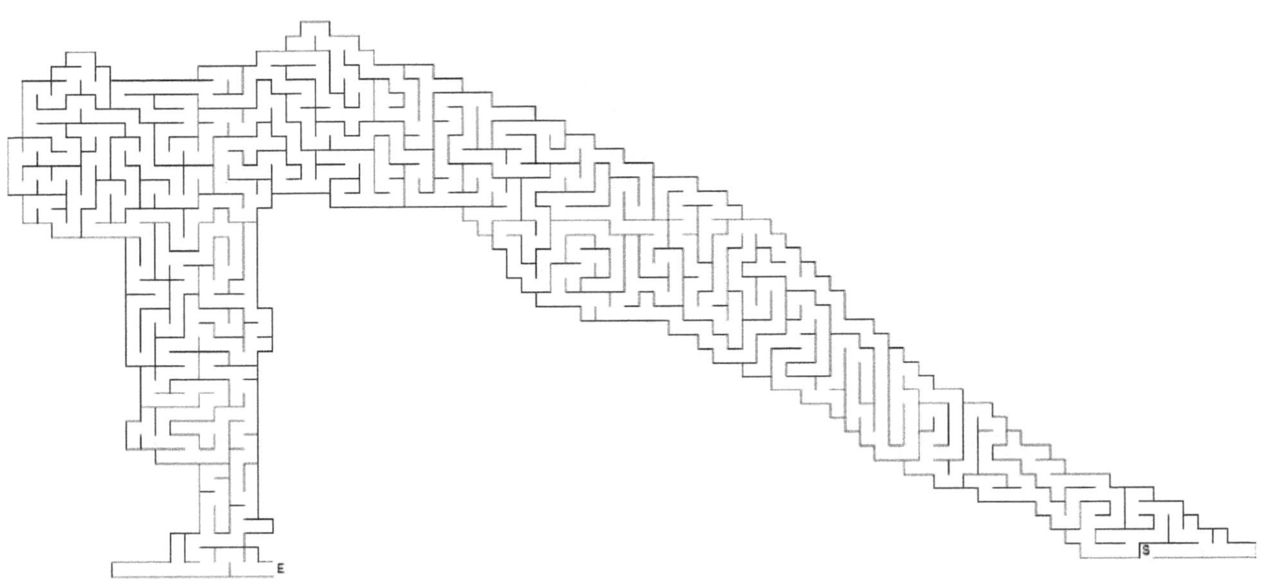

Sudoku #36

★★★★

Sudoku #37

★★★★★

Yoga
Maze #37

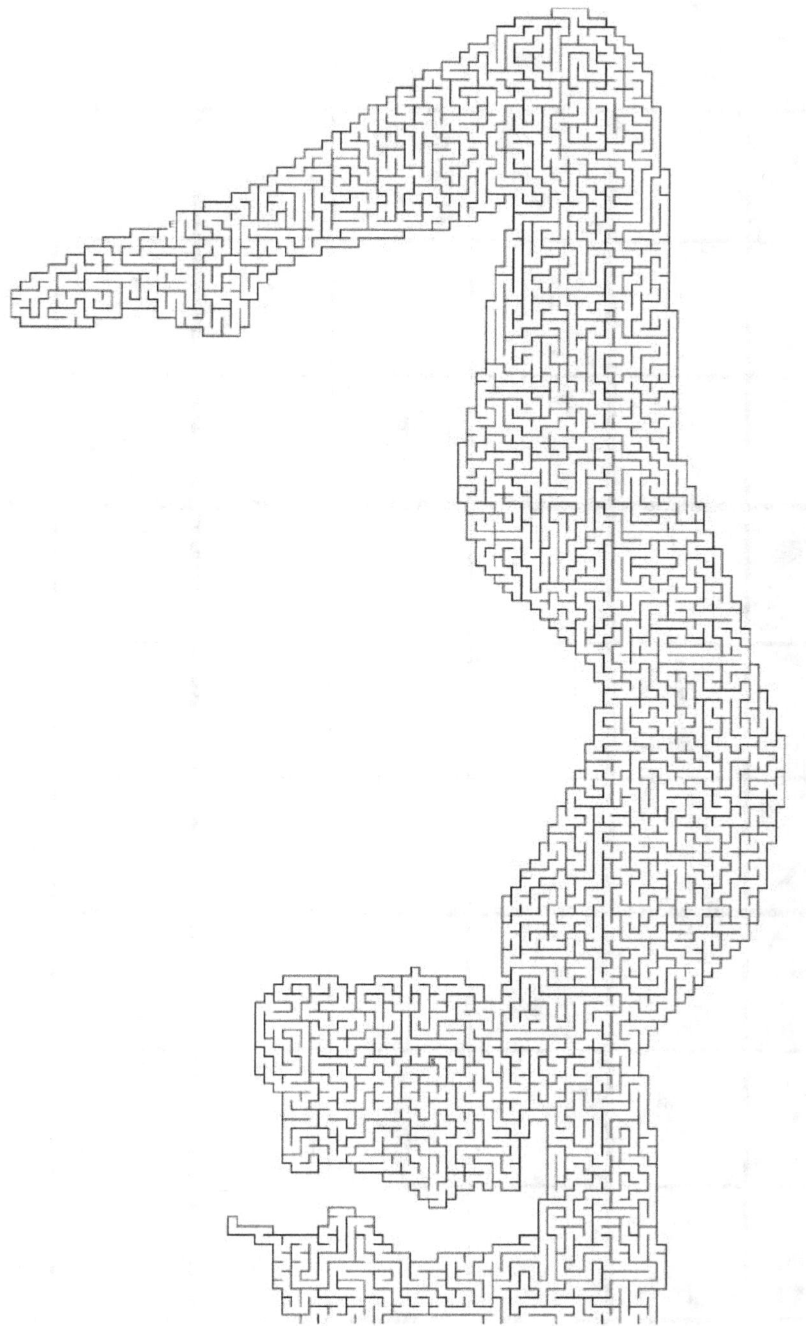

Sudoku #38

Yoga
Maze #38

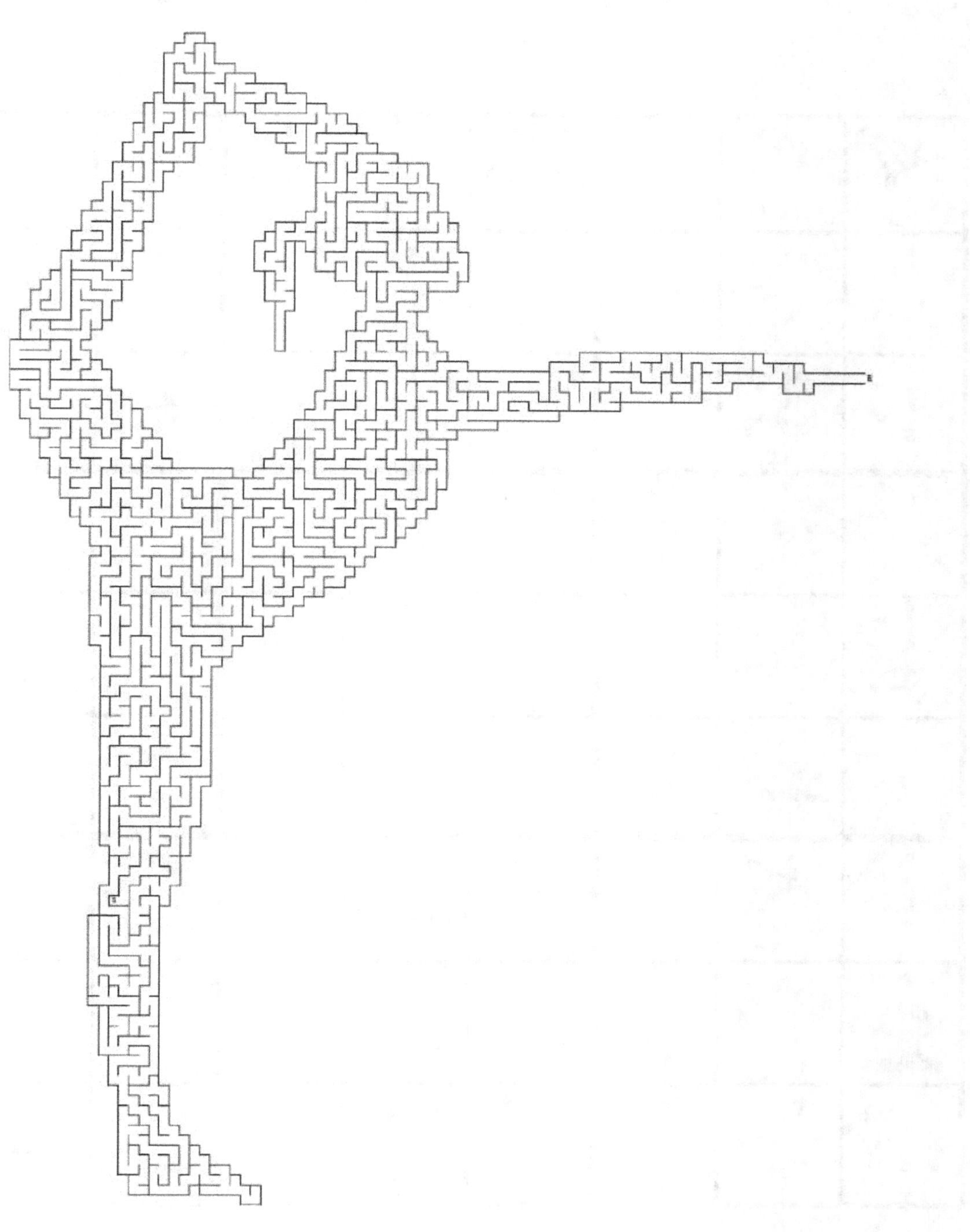

Sudoku #39

★ ★ ★ ★

Yoga
Maze #39

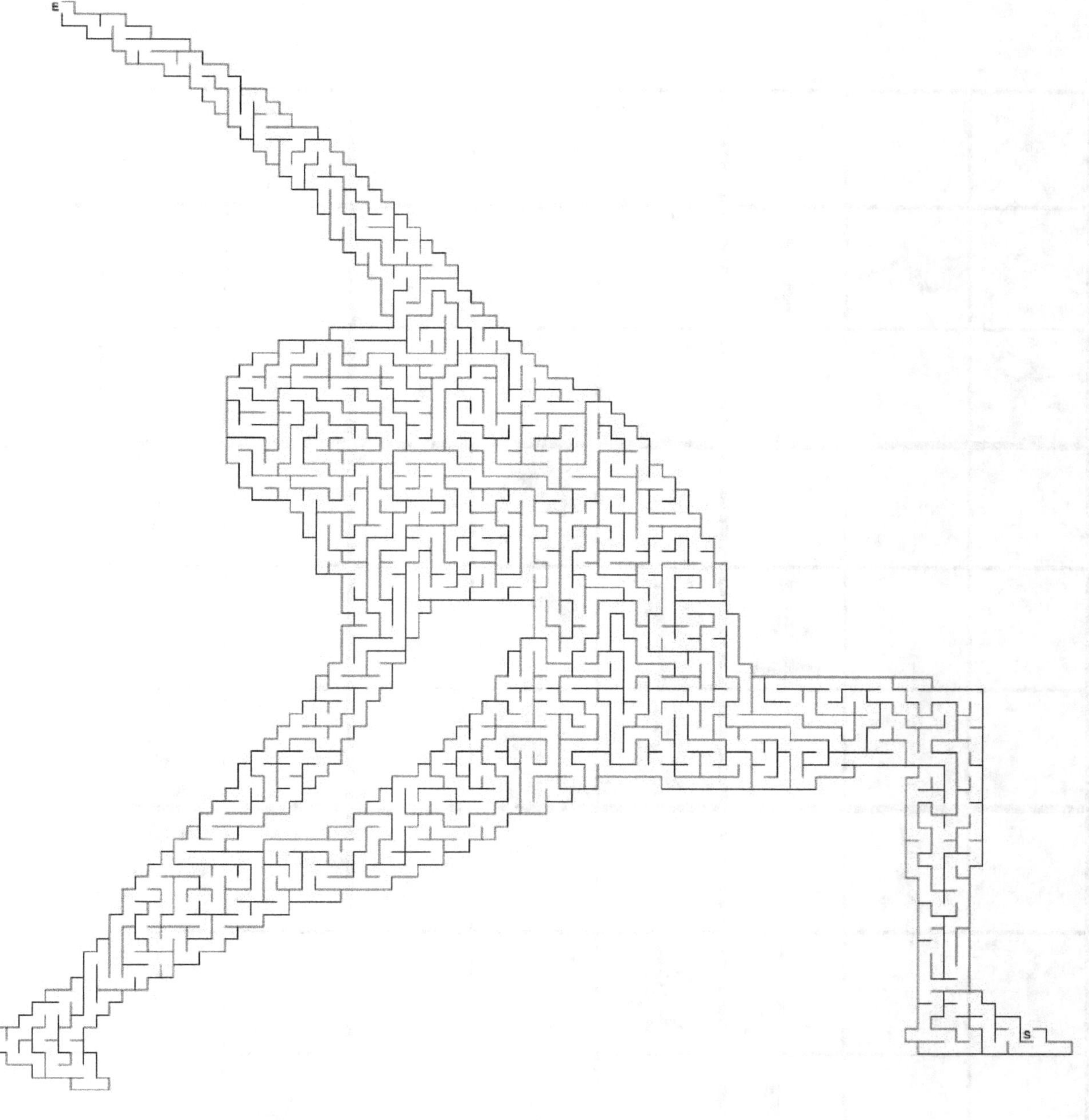

Sudoku #40

★★★★

Yoga
Maze #40

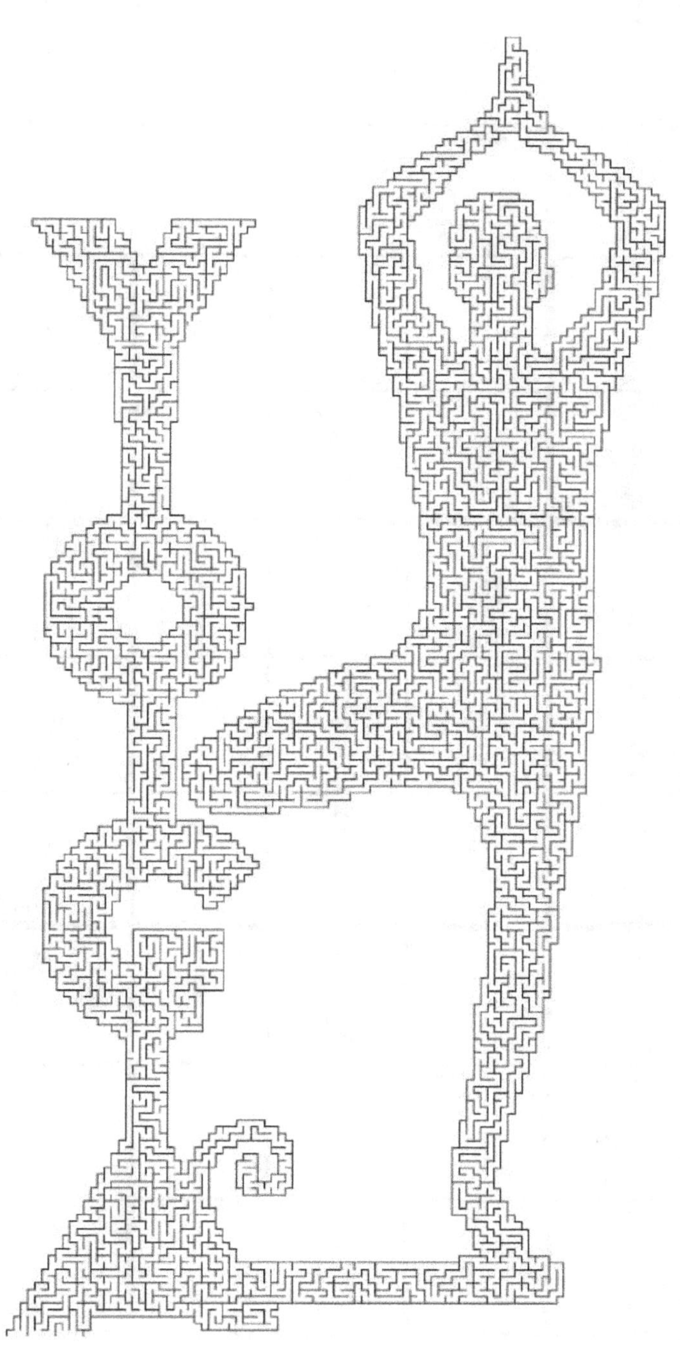

Sudoku #41

★★★★★

Sudoku #42

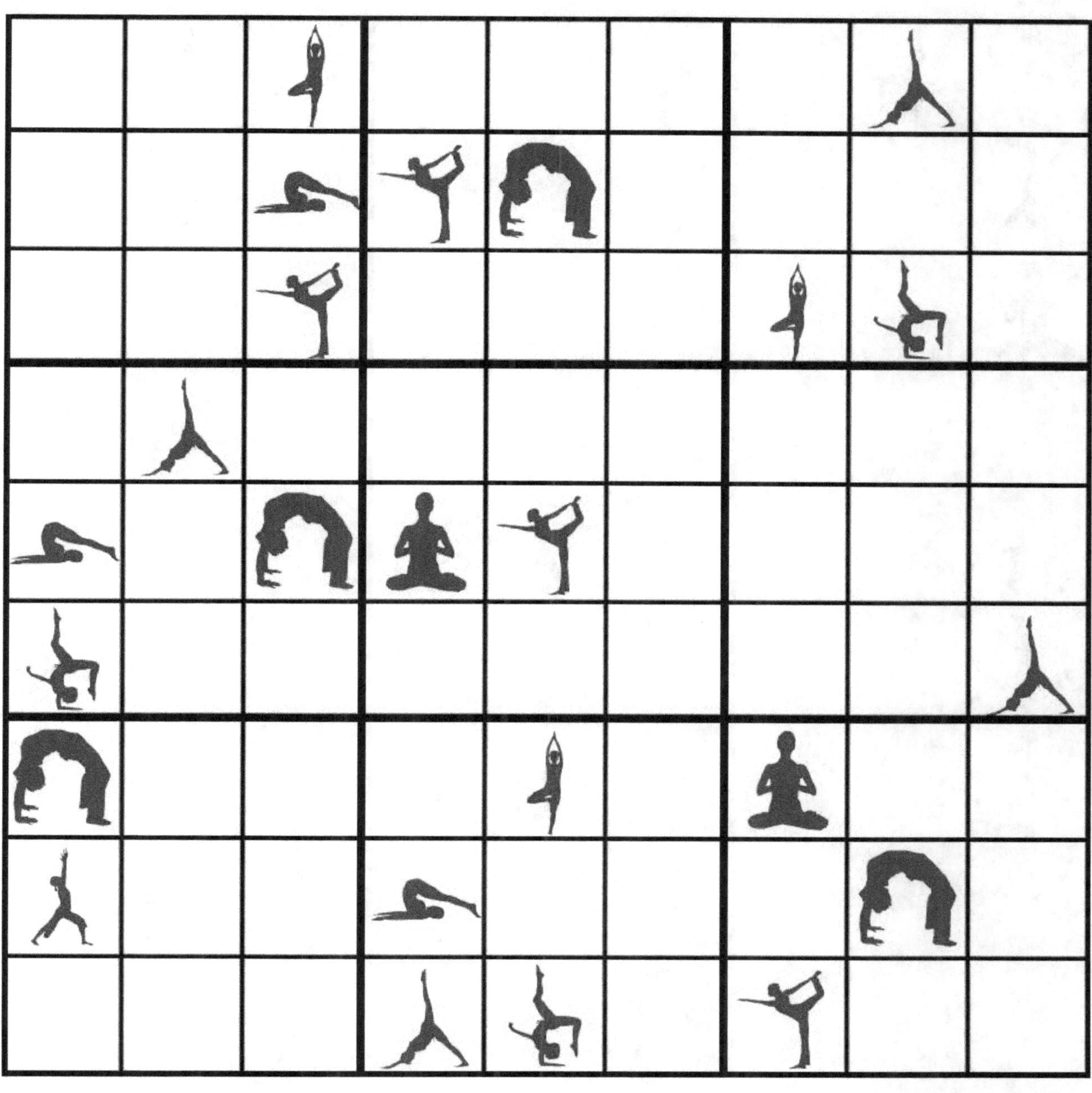

Sudoku #43

★★★★★

Sudoku #44

★ ★ ★ ★ ★

Sudoku #45

★★★★★

Sudoku #46

★★★★★

Sudoku #47

★★★★★

Sudoku #48

Sudoku #49

★★★★★

Sudoku #50

★ ★ ★ ★ ★

Sudoku #51

★★★★★★

Sudoku #52

Sudoku #53

★★★★★★

Sudoku #54

Sudoku #55

Sudoku #56

Sudoku #57

Sudoku #58

★ ★ ★ ★ ★ ★

Sudoku #59

★ ★ ★ ★ ★ ★

Sudoku #60

Answers

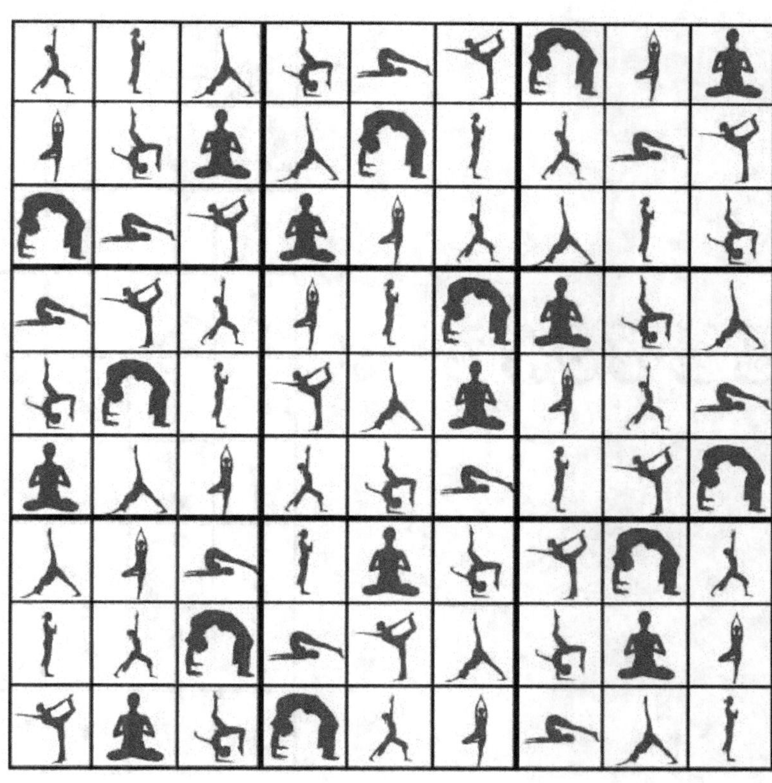

Sudoku 1

Sudoku 2

Sudoku 3

Sudoku 4

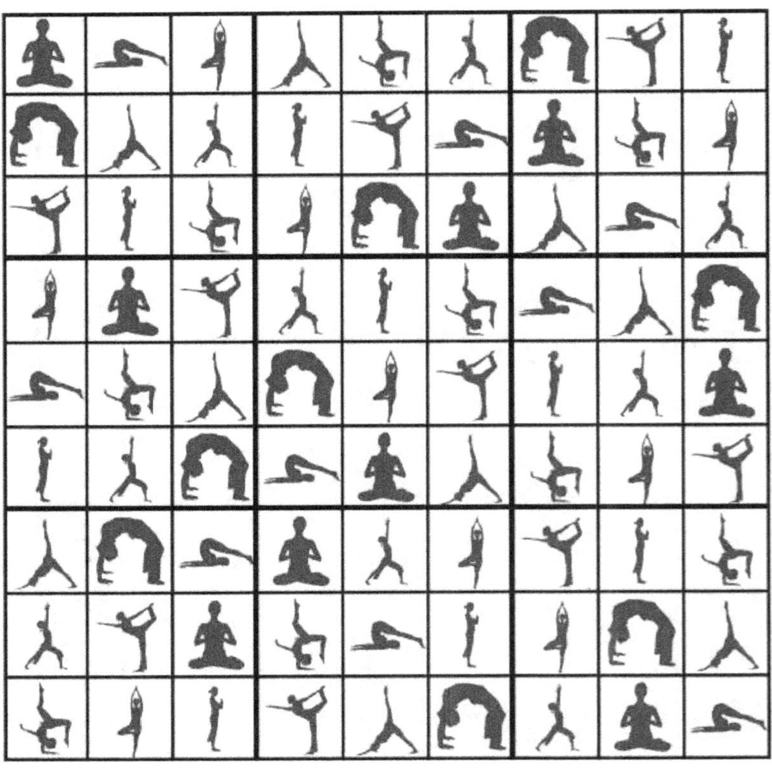

Sudoku 5

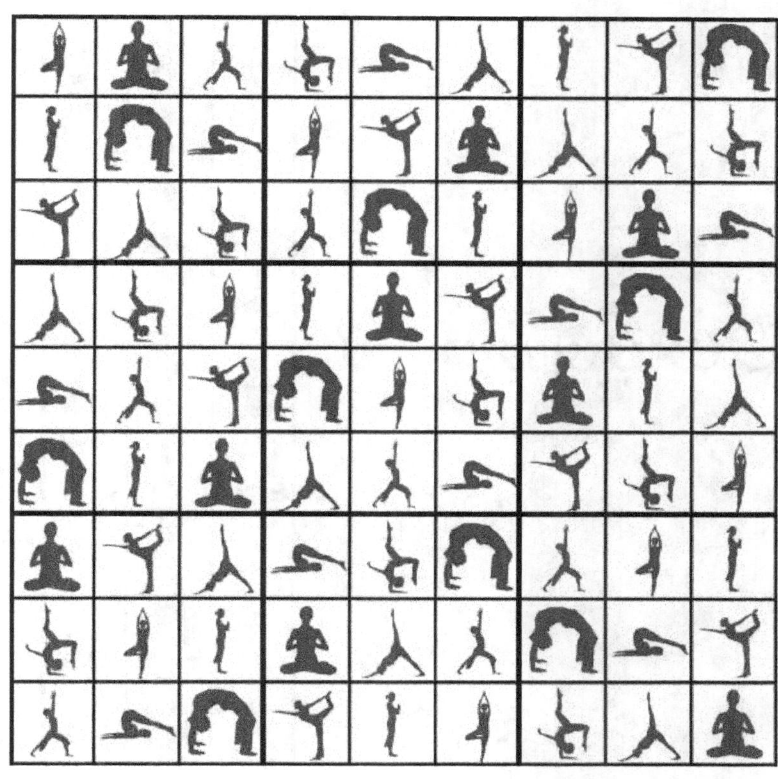

Sudoku 6

Sudoku 7

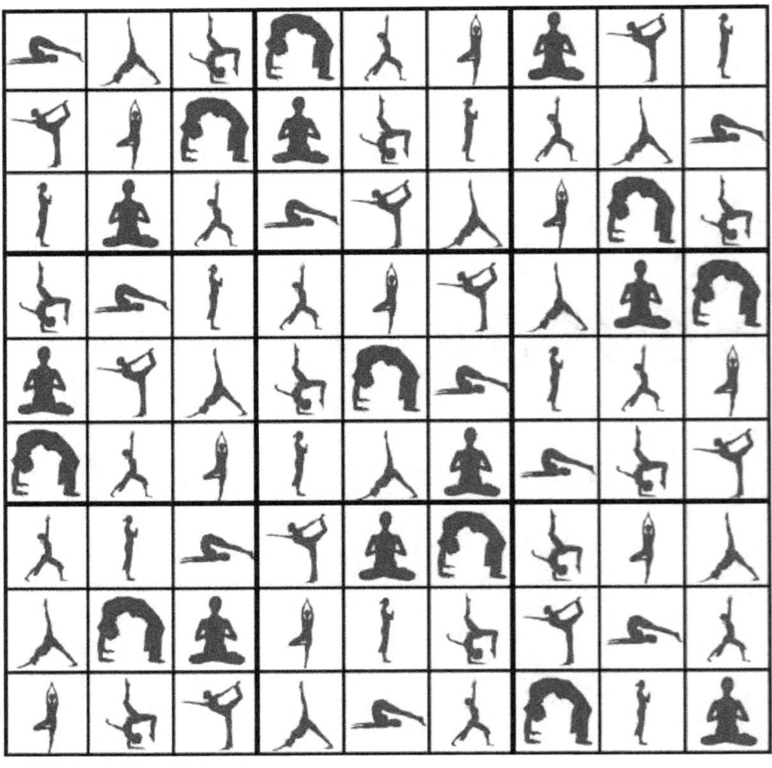

Sudoku 8

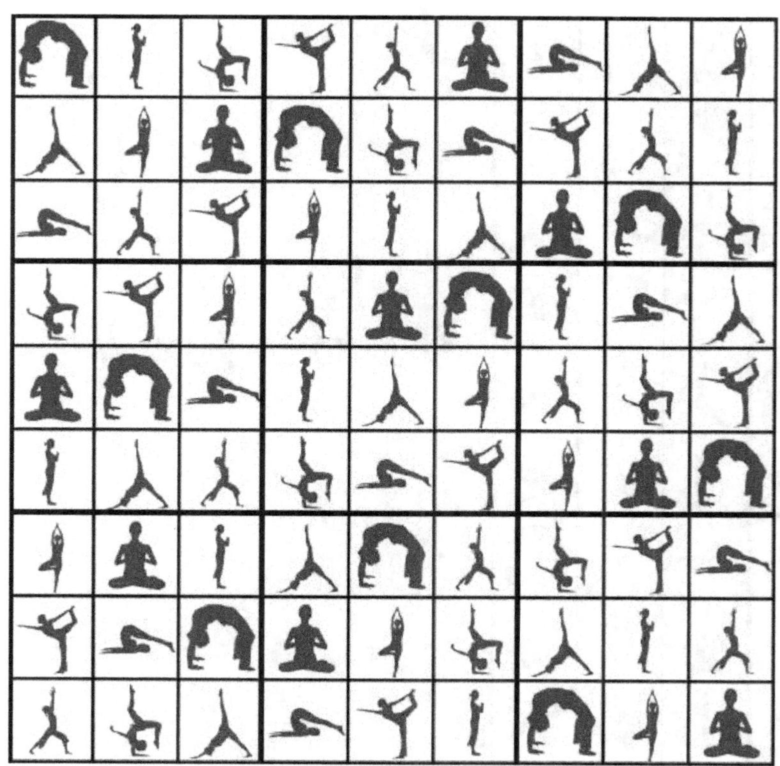

Sudoku 9

Sudoku 10

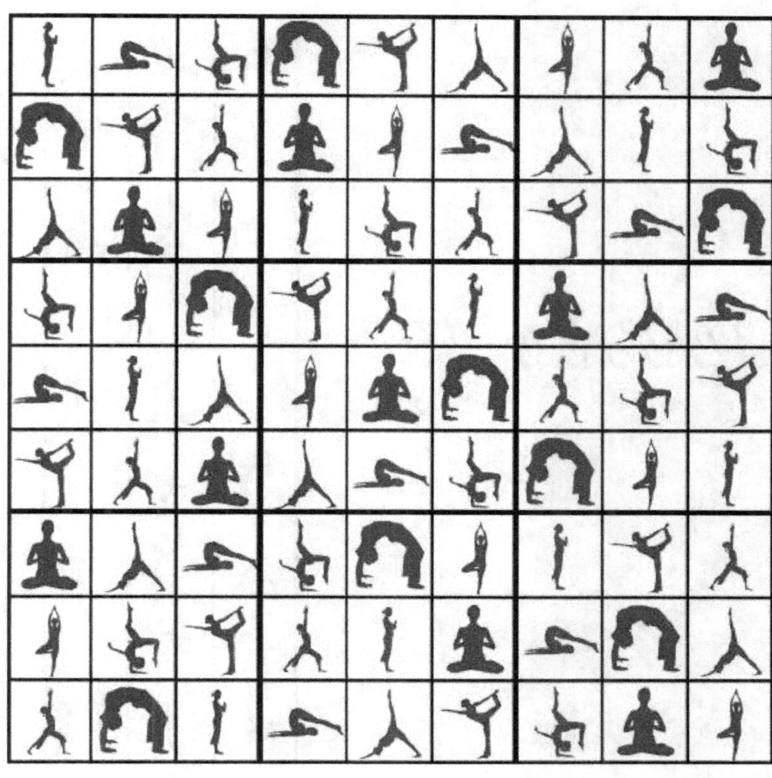

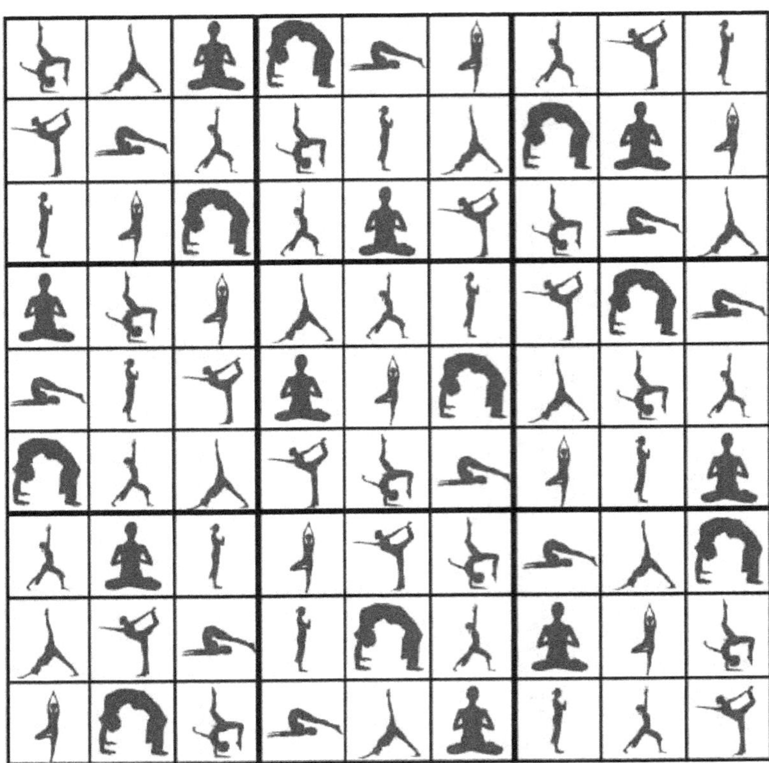

Sudoku 11

Sudoku 12

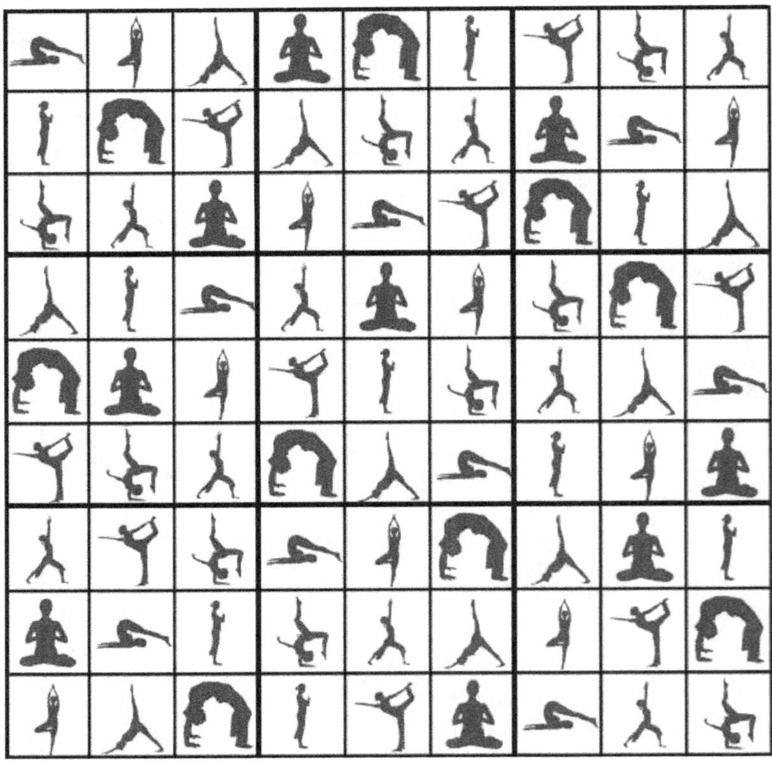

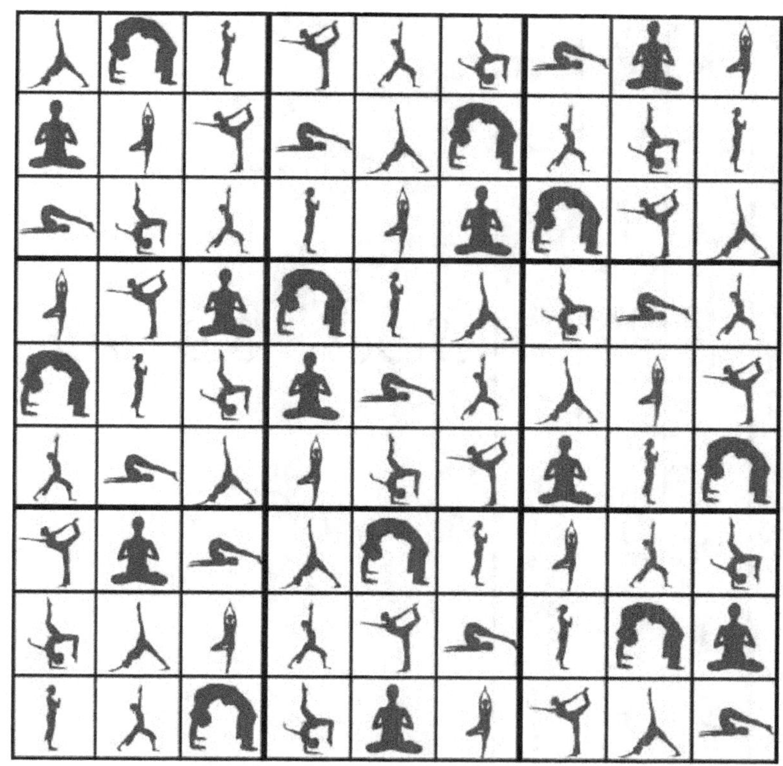

Sudoku 13

Sudoku 14

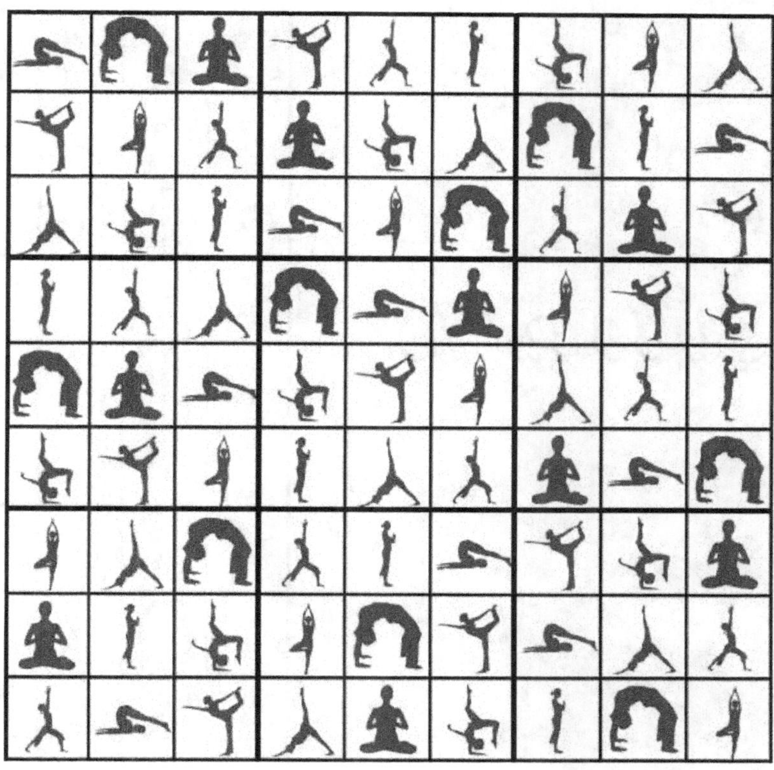

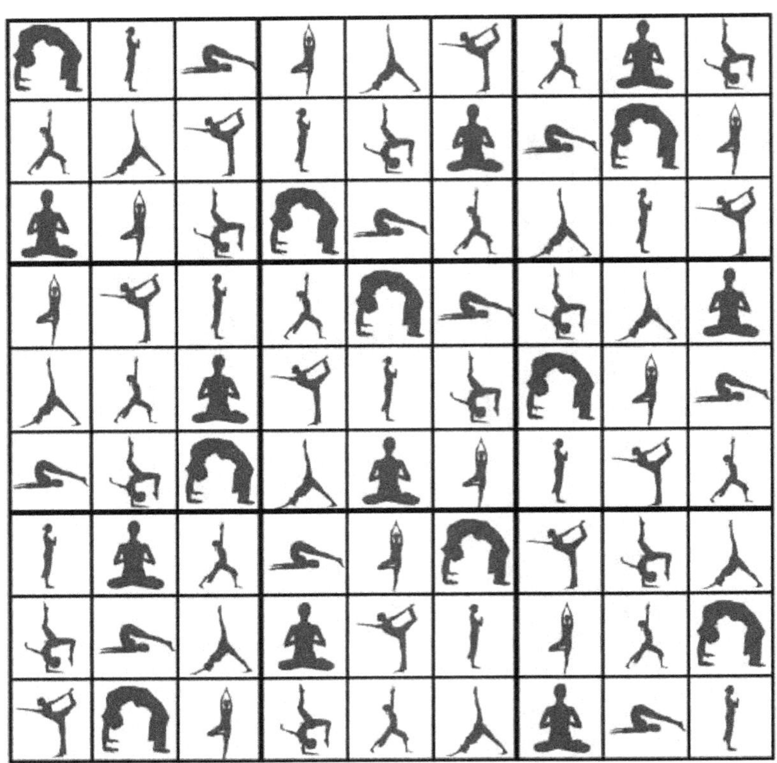

Sudoku 15

Sudoku 16

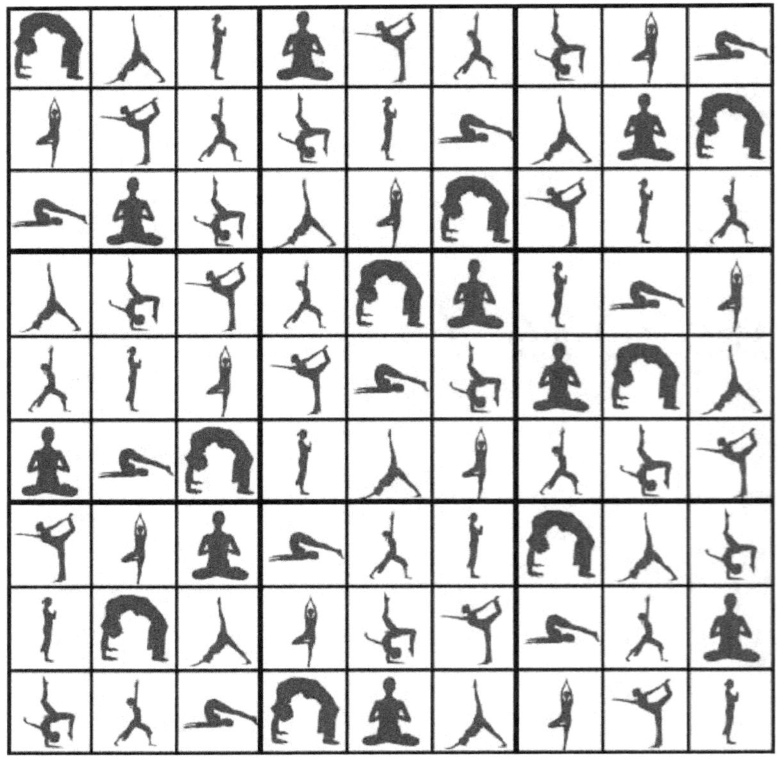

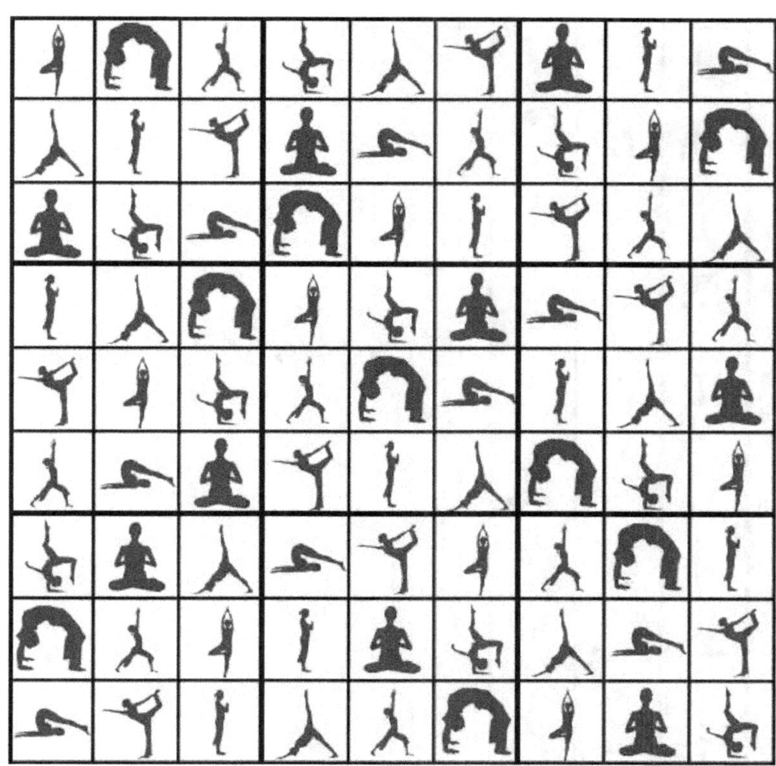

Sudoku 17

Sudoku 18

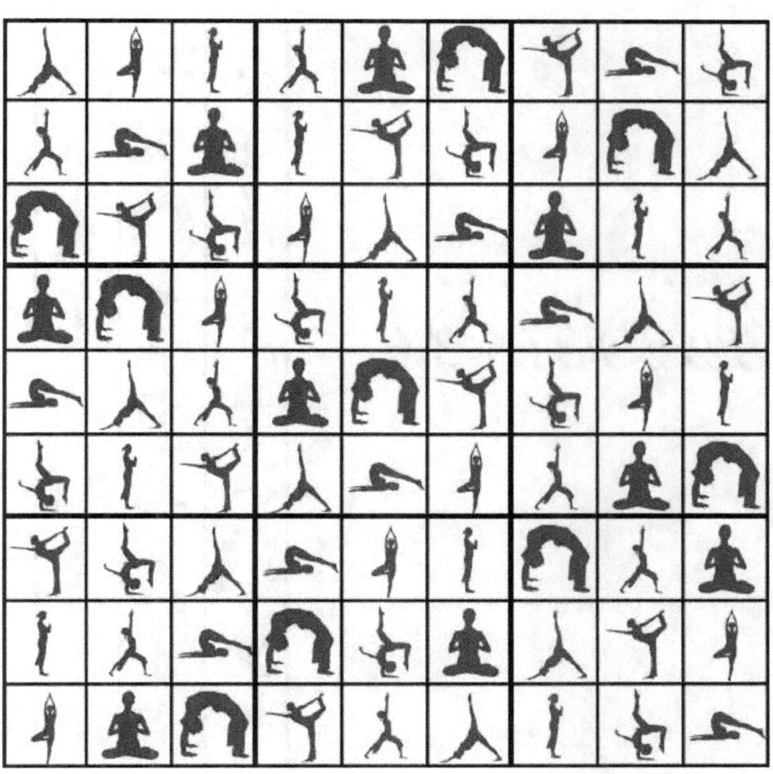

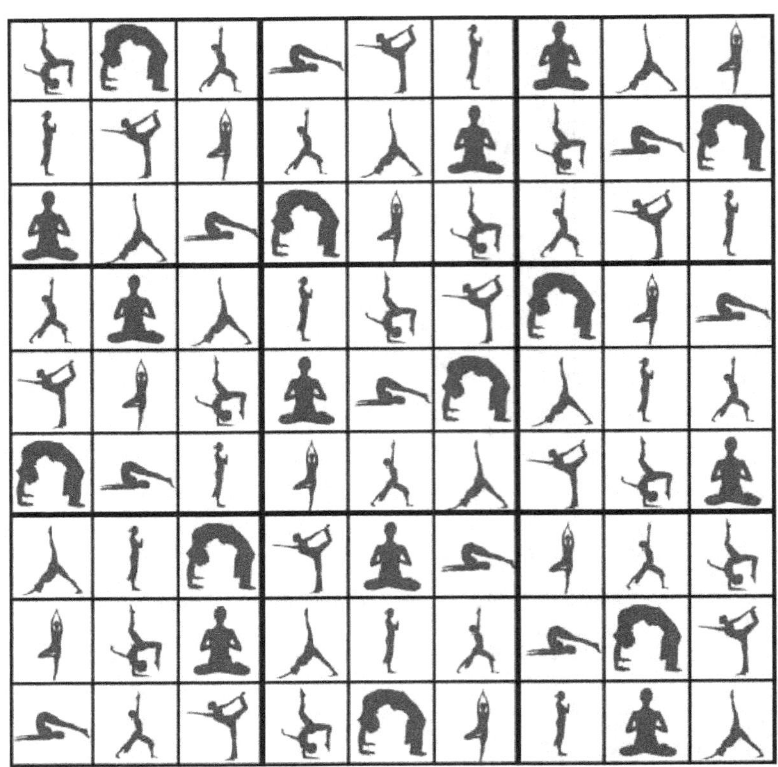

Sudoku 19

Sudoku 20

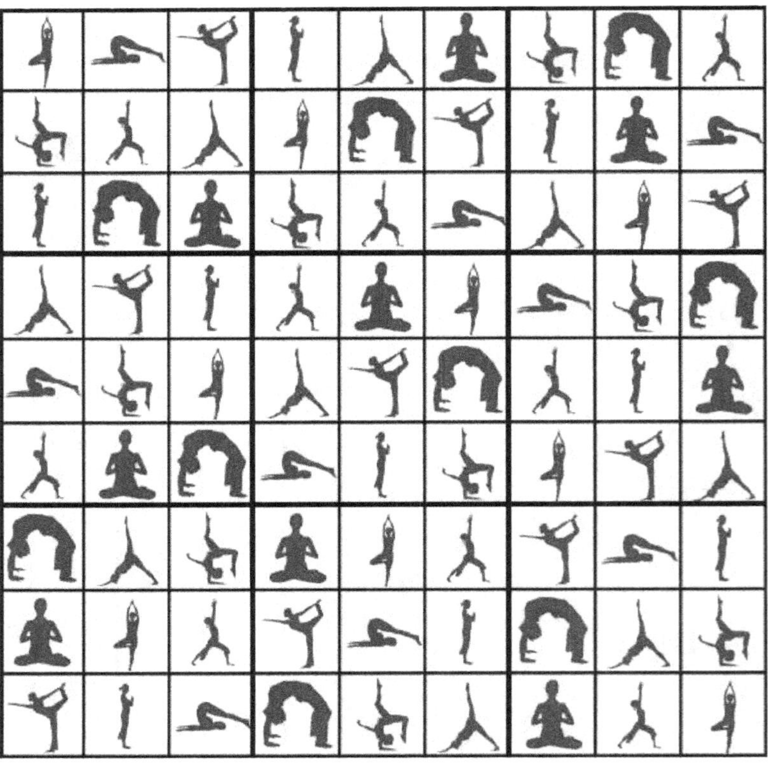

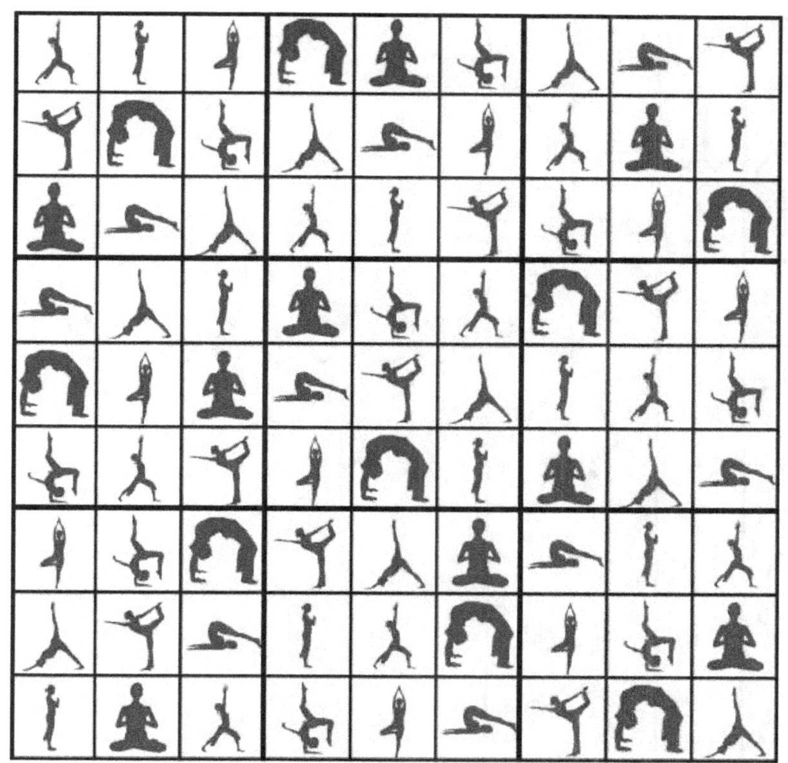

Sudoku 21

Sudoku 22

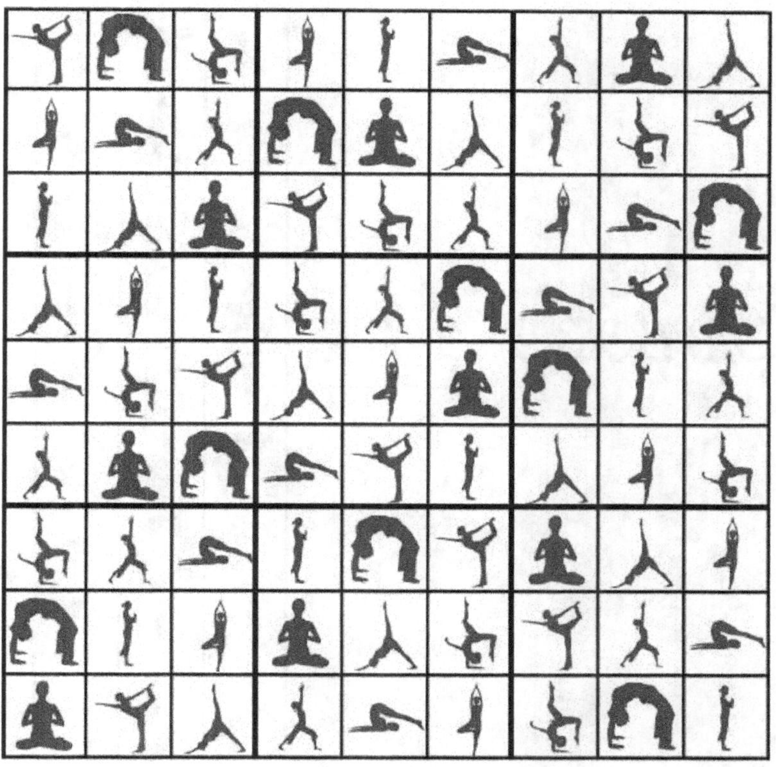

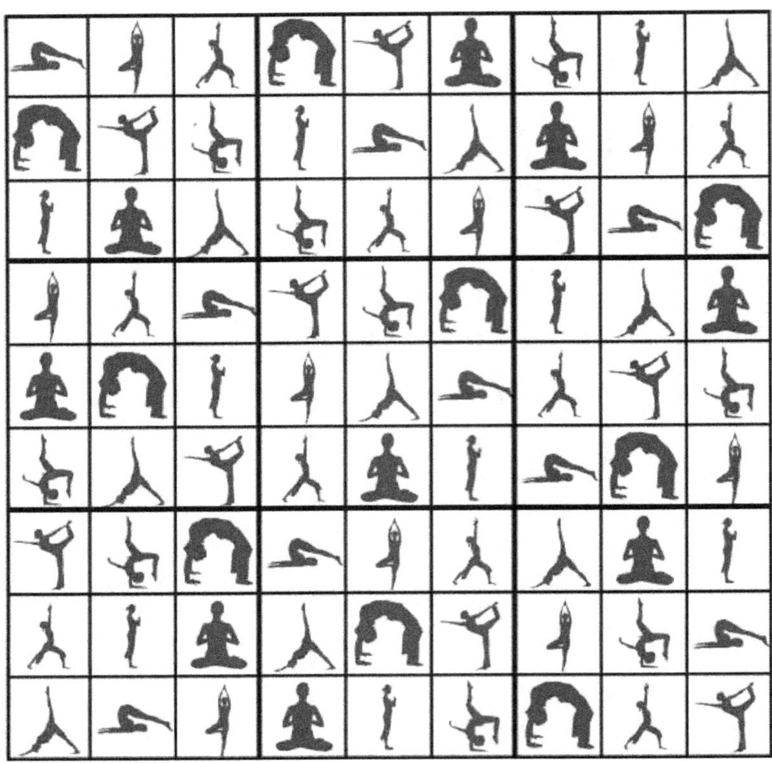

Sudoku 23

Sudoku 24

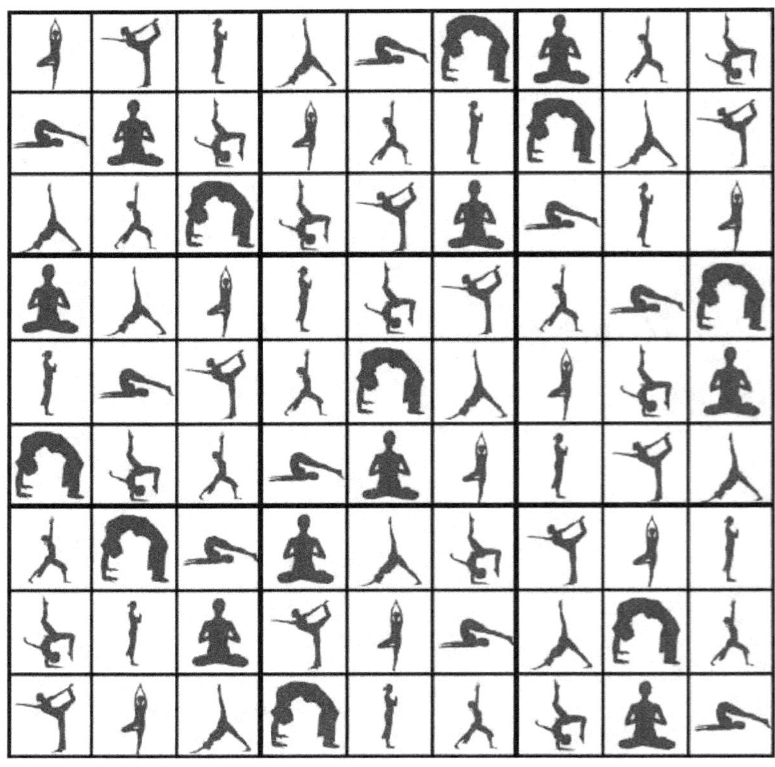

Sudoku 25

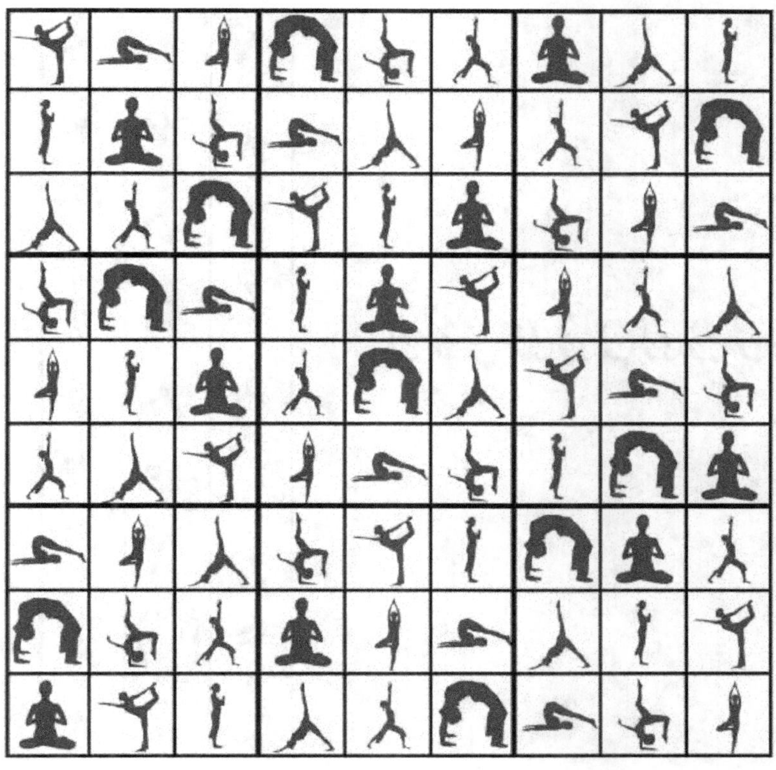

Sudoku 26

Sudoku 27

Sudoku 28

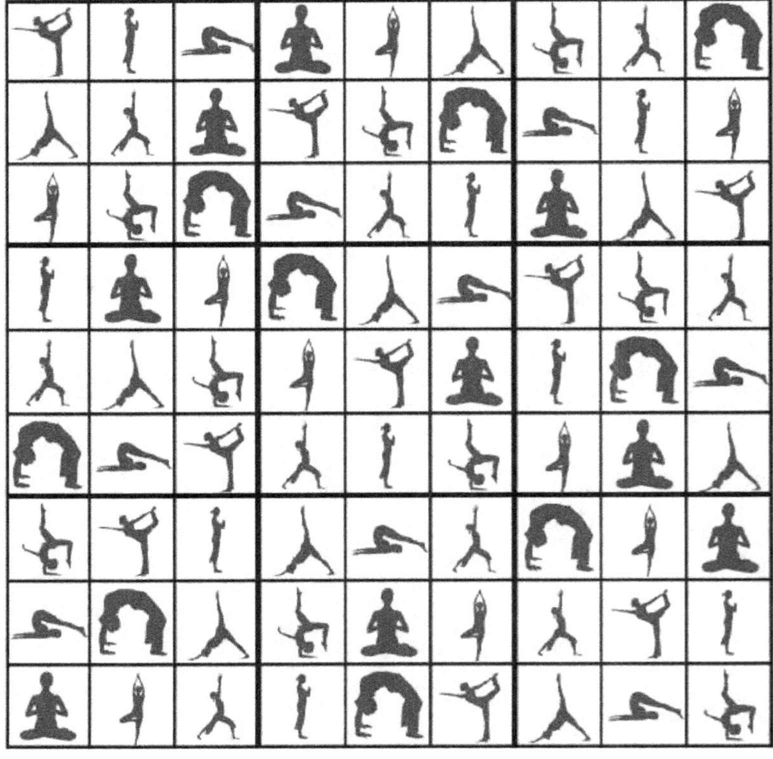

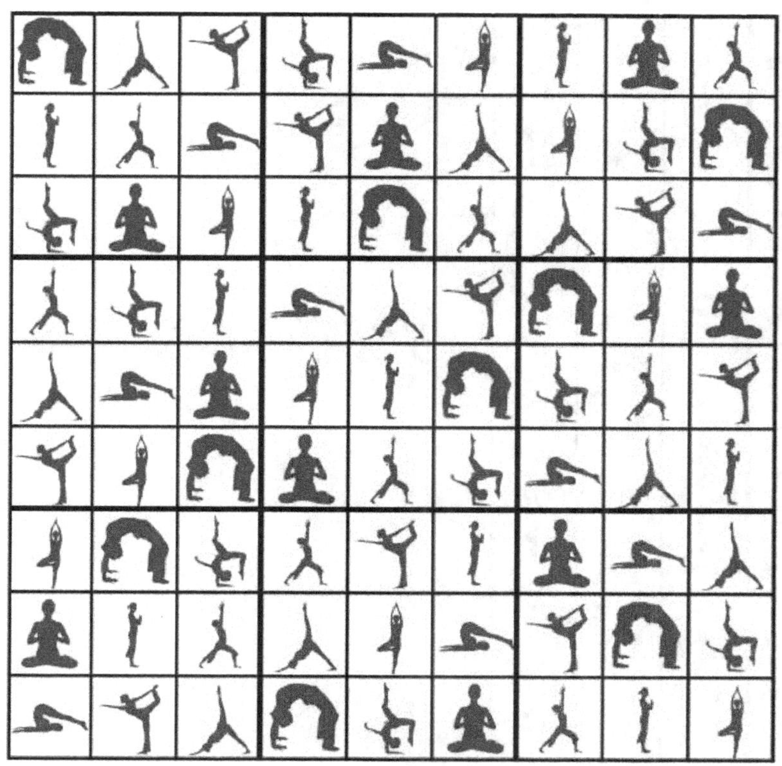

Sudoku 29

Sudoku 30

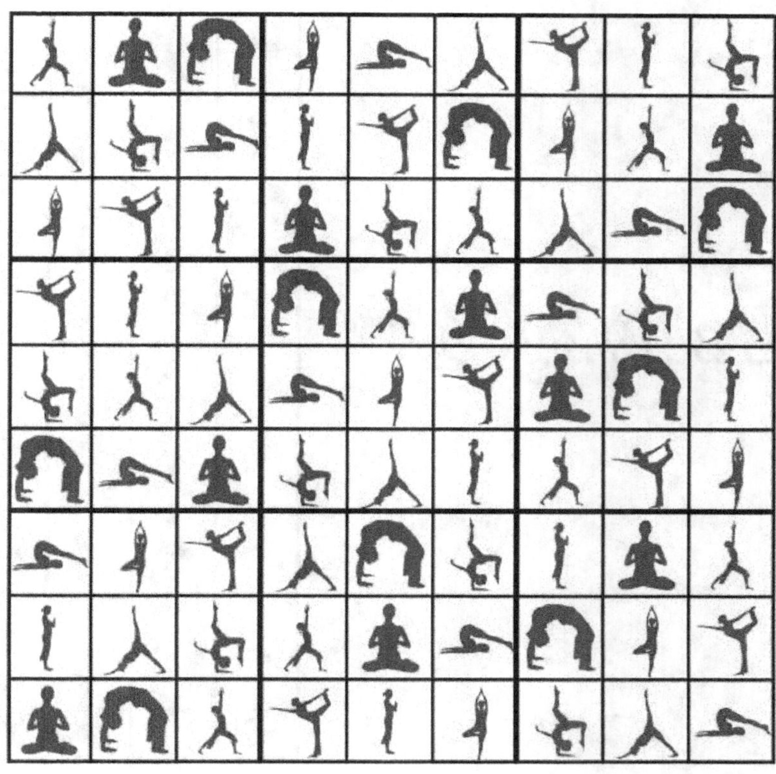

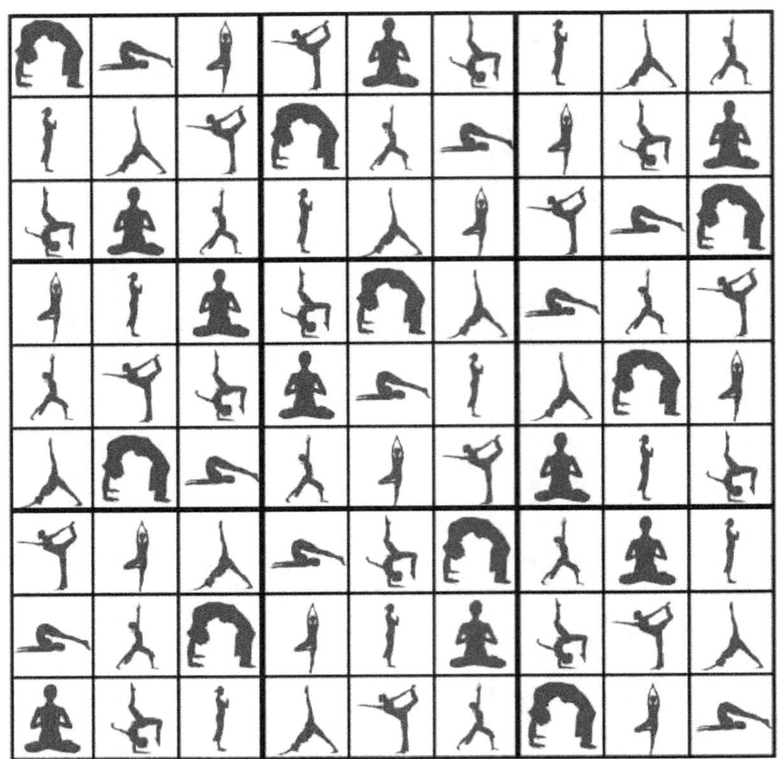

Sudoku 31

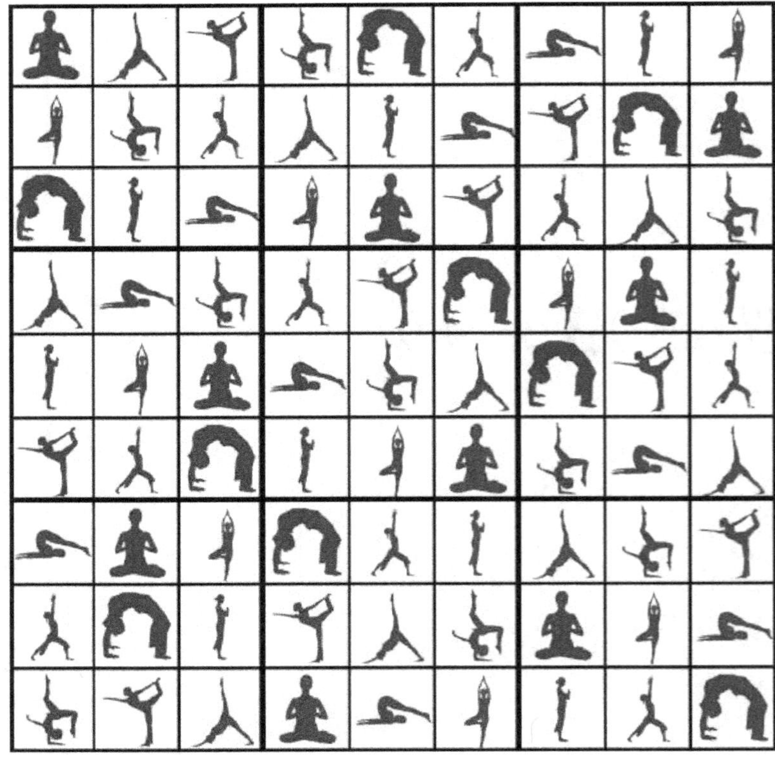

Sudoku 32

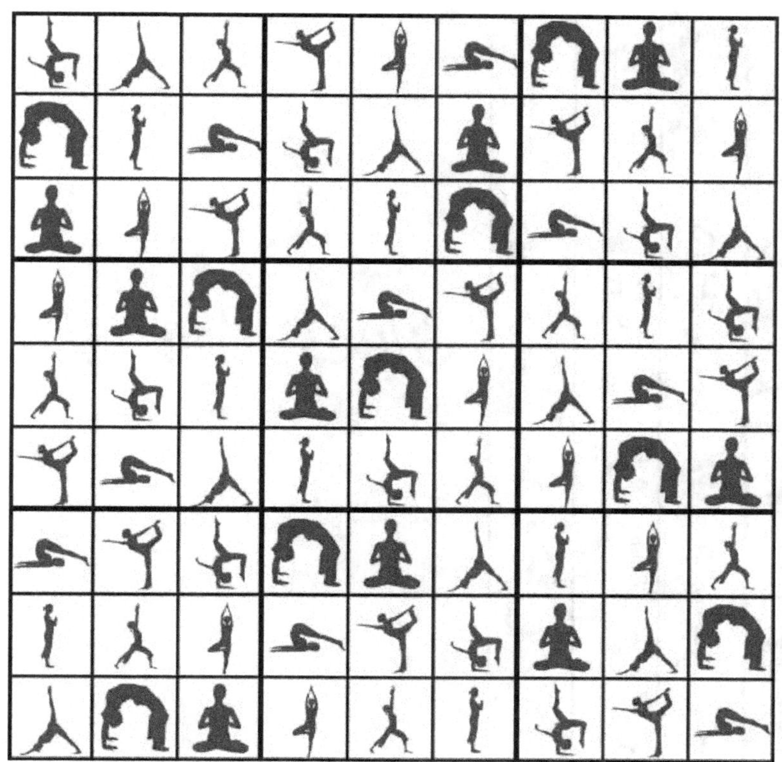

Sudoku 33

Sudoku 34

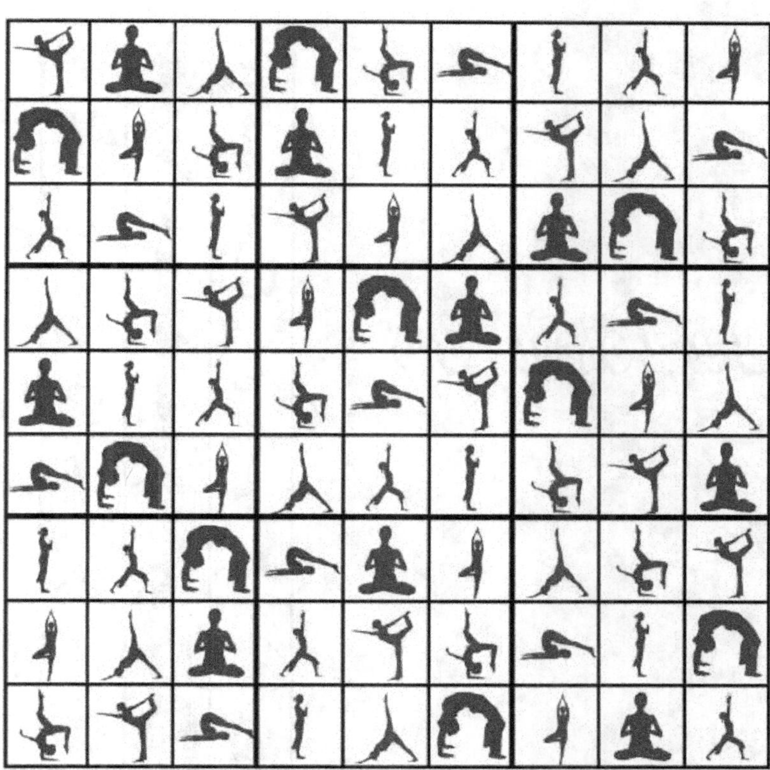

Sudoku 35

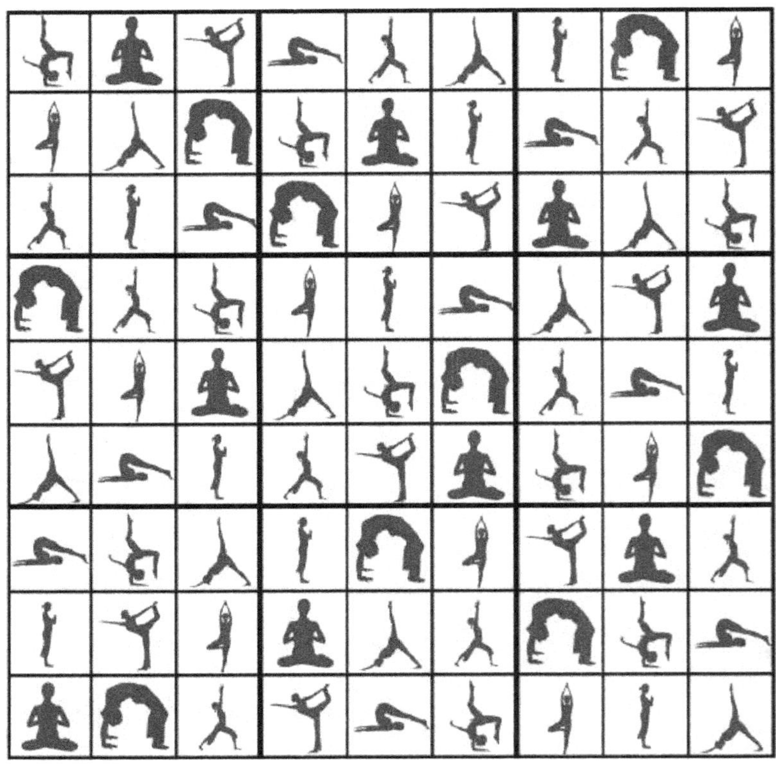

Sudoku 36

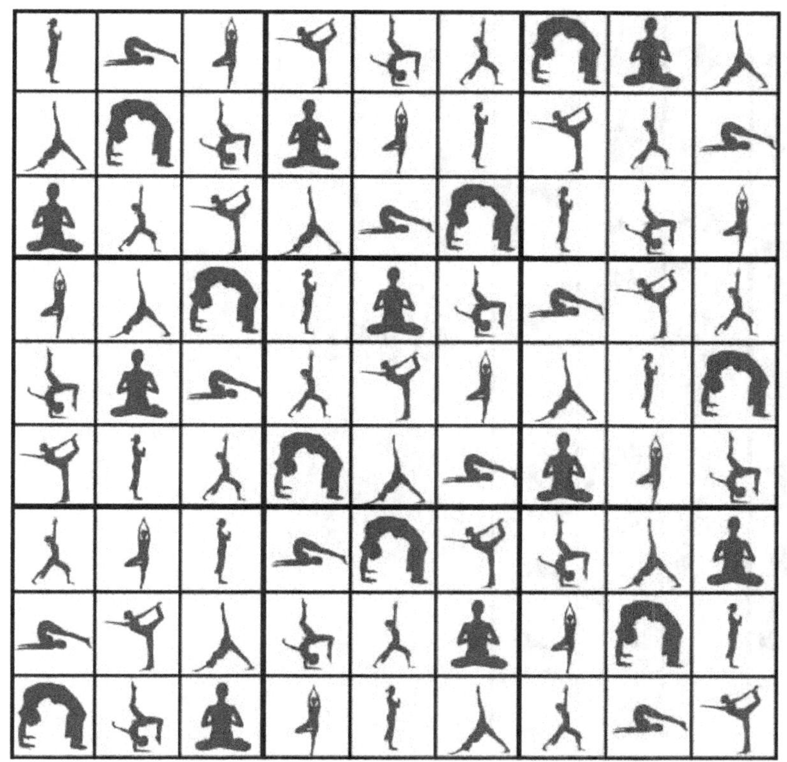

Sudoku 37

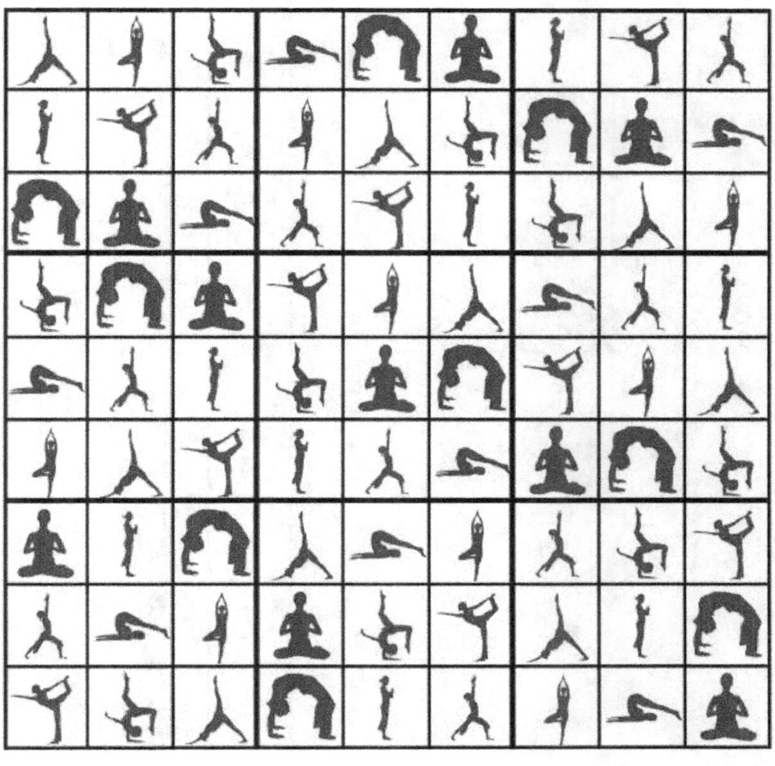

Sudoku 38

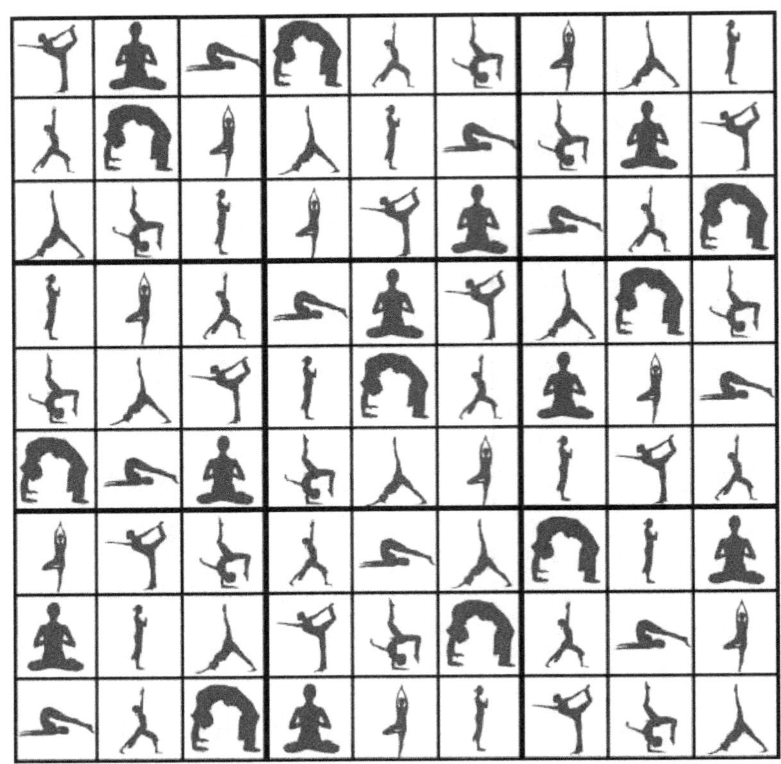

Sudoku 39

Sudoku 40

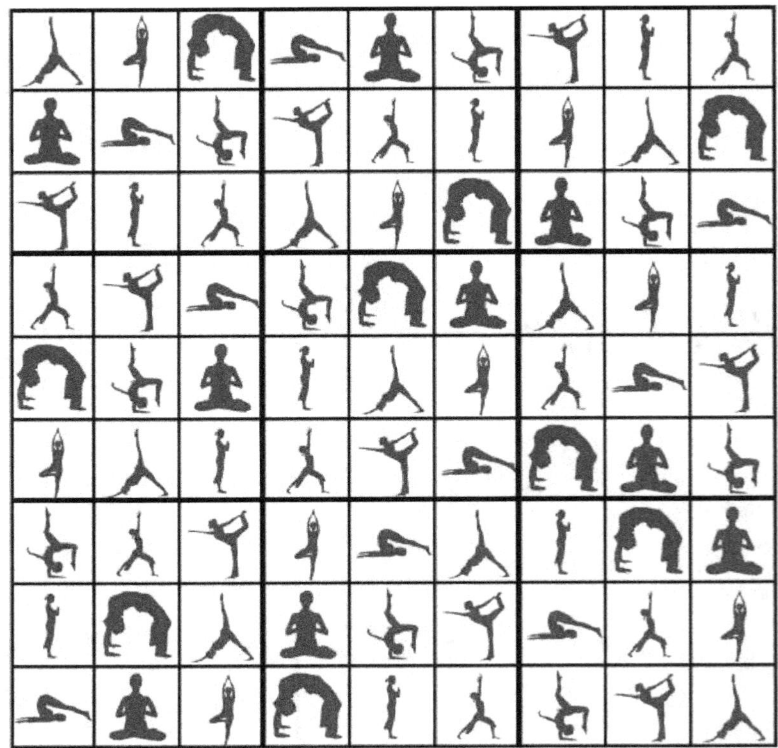

Sudoku 41

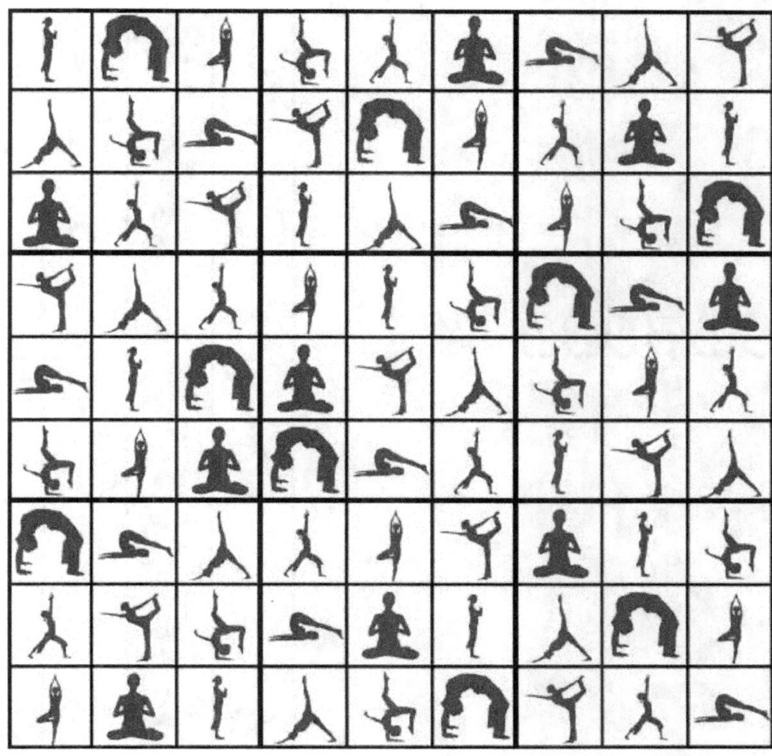

Sudoku 42

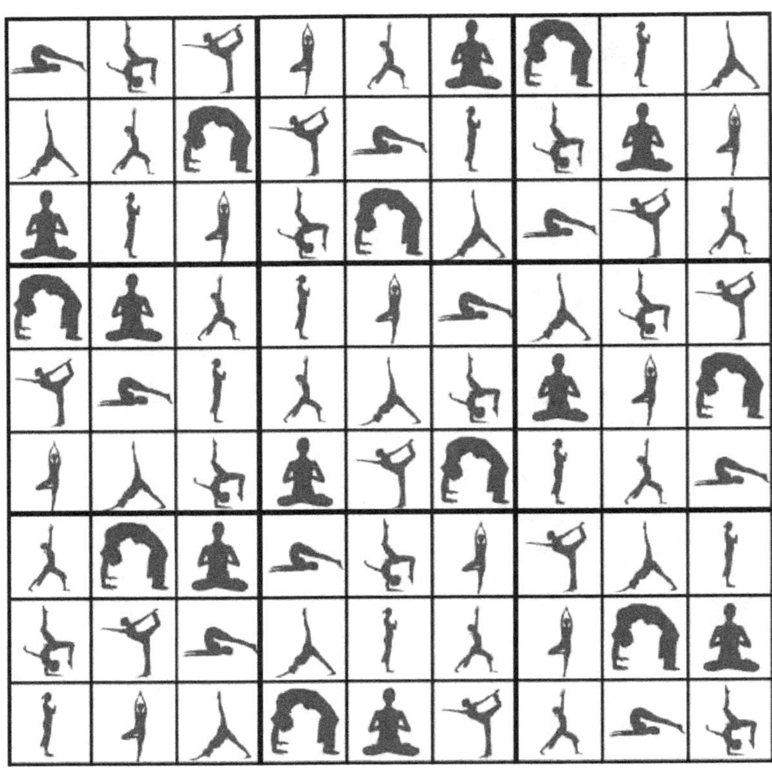

Sudoku 43

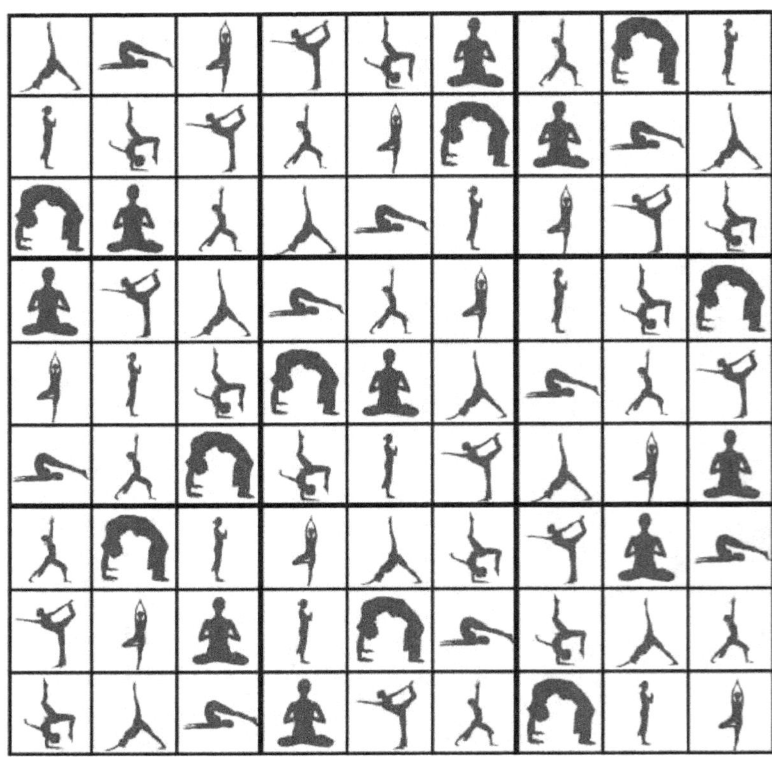

Sudoku 44

Sudoku 45

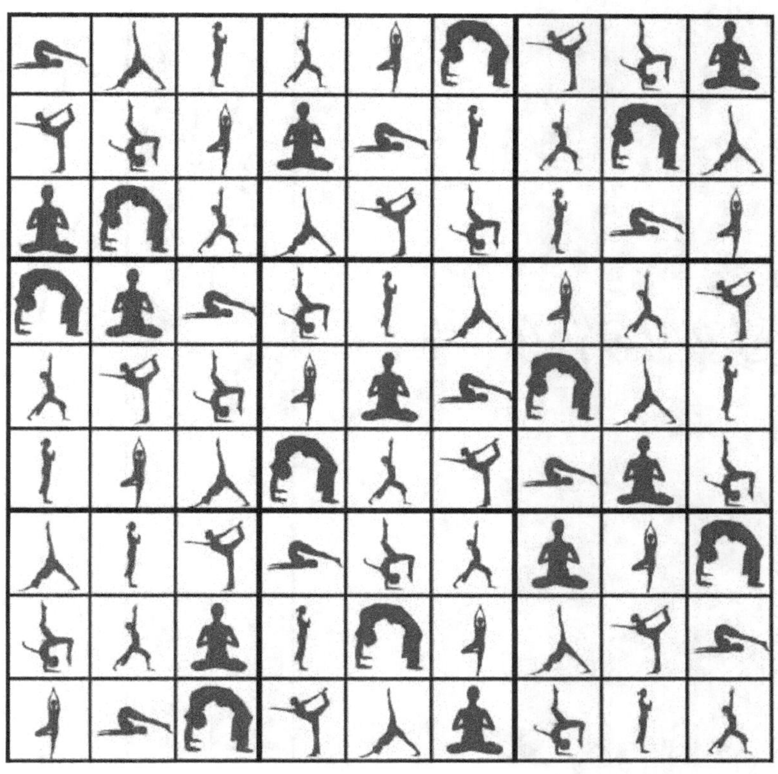

Sudoku 46

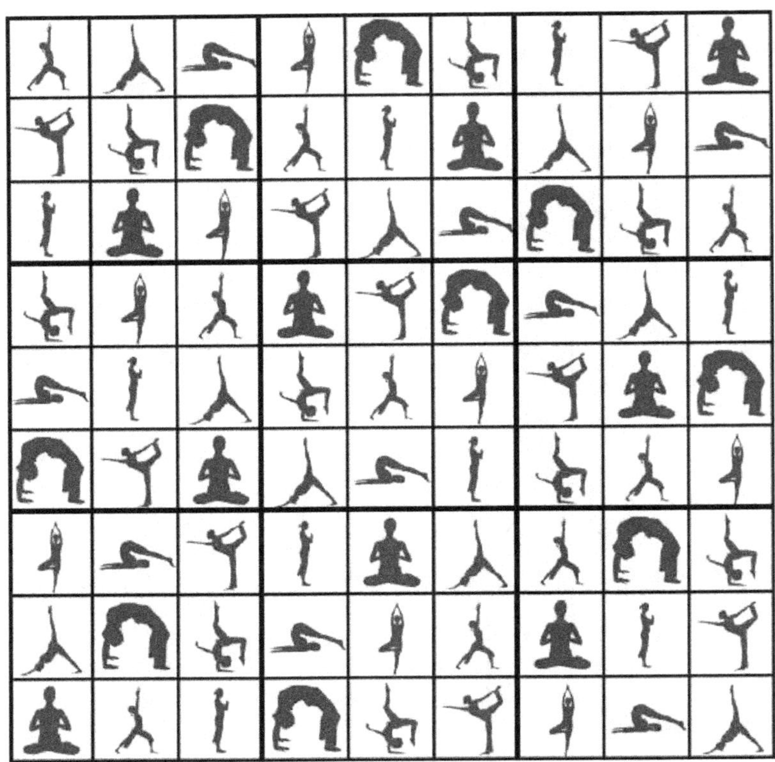

Sudoku 47

Sudoku 48

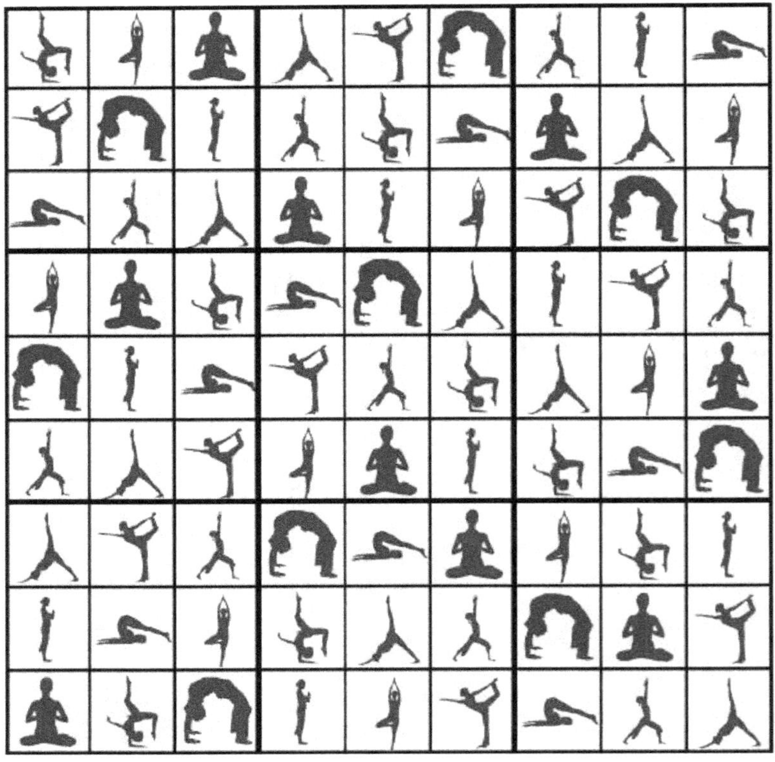

Sudoku 49

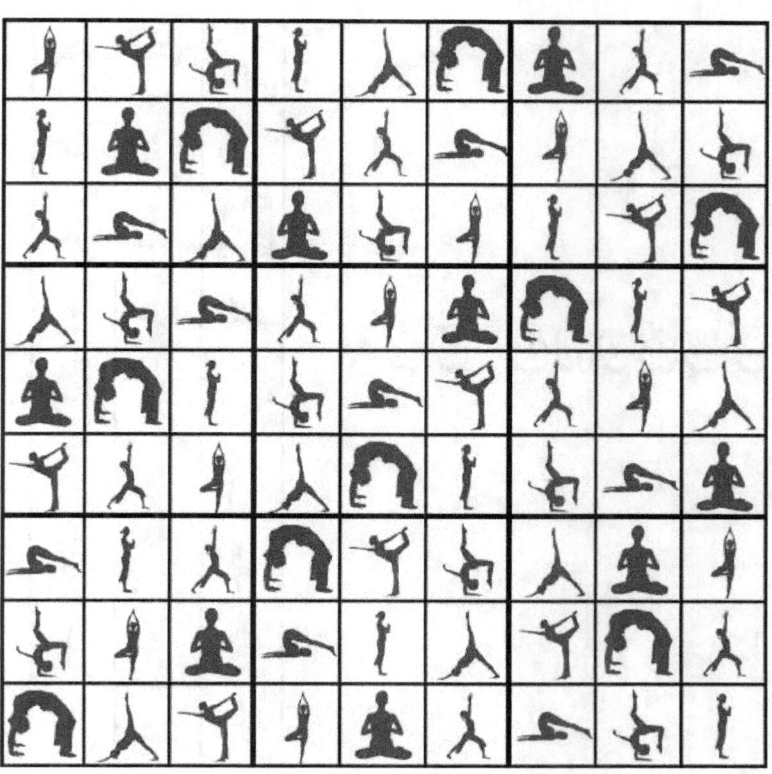

Sudoku 50

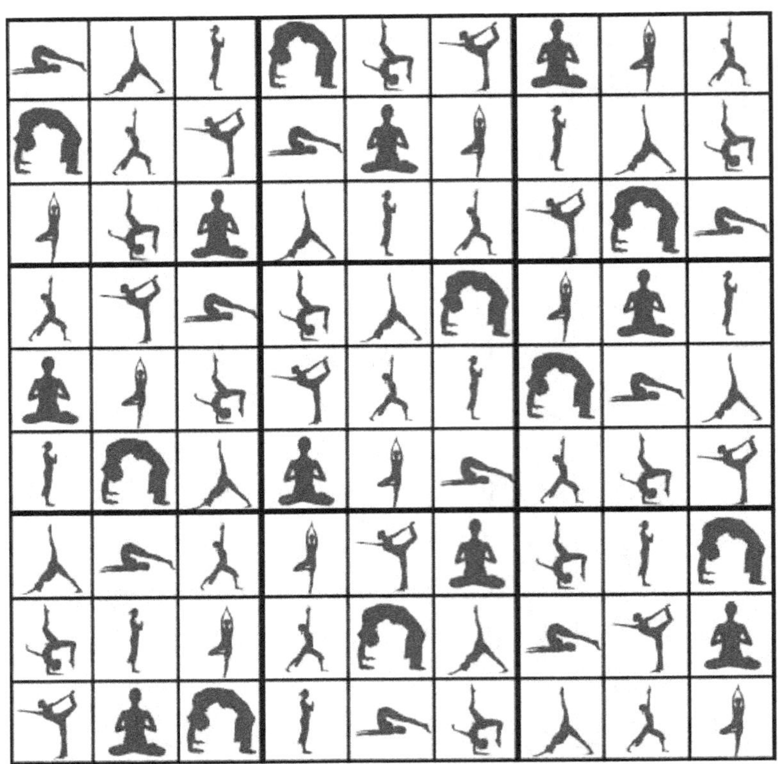

Sudoku 51

Sudoku 52

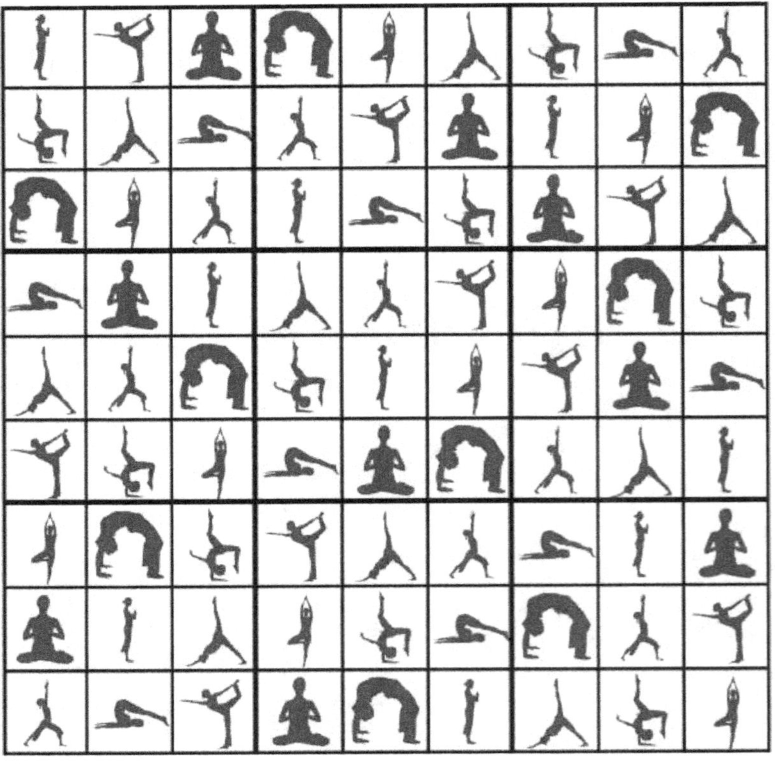

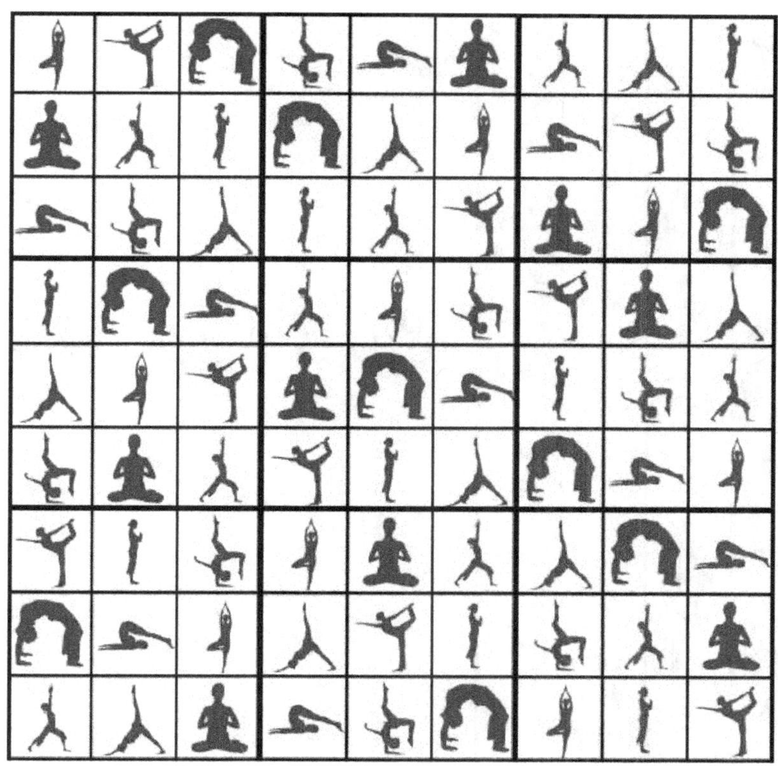

Sudoku 53

Sudoku 54

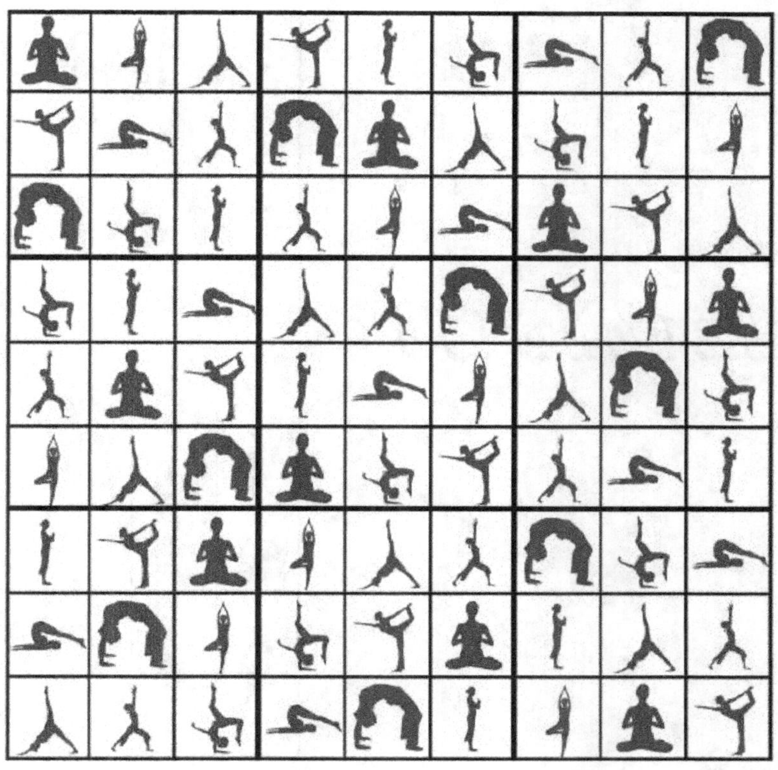

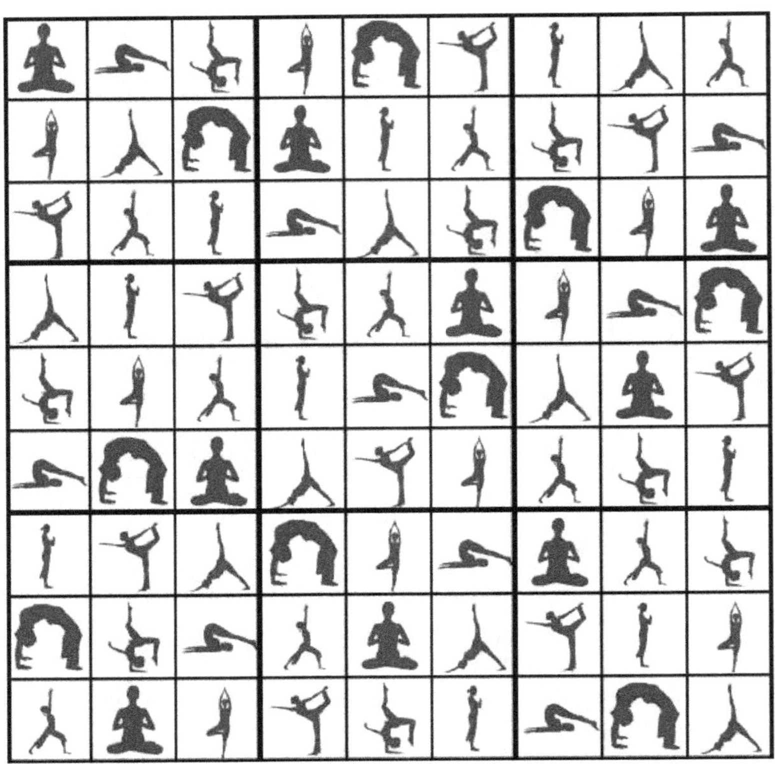

Sudoku 55

Sudoku 56

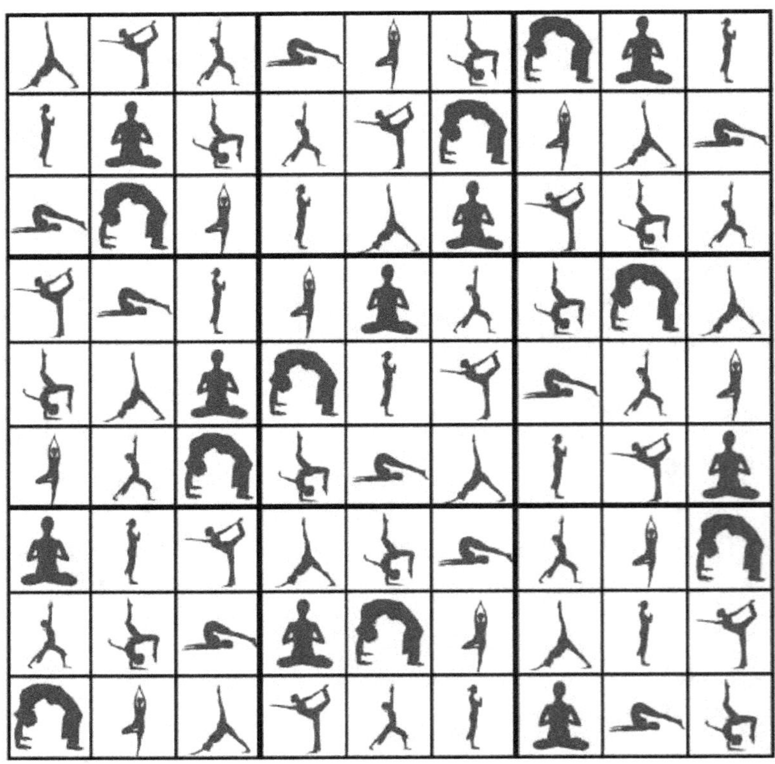

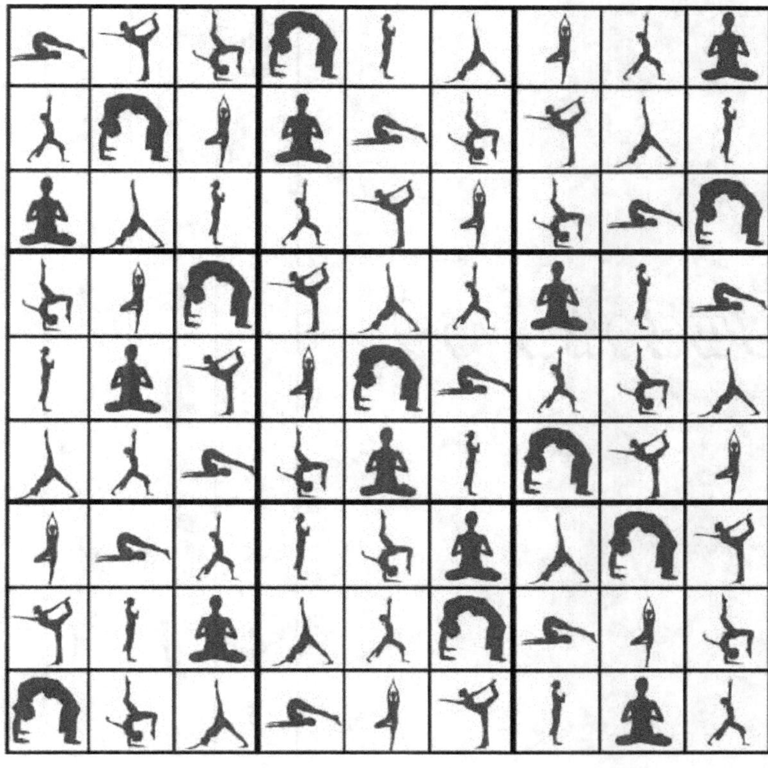

Sudoku 57

Sudoku 58

Sudoku 59

Sudoku 60

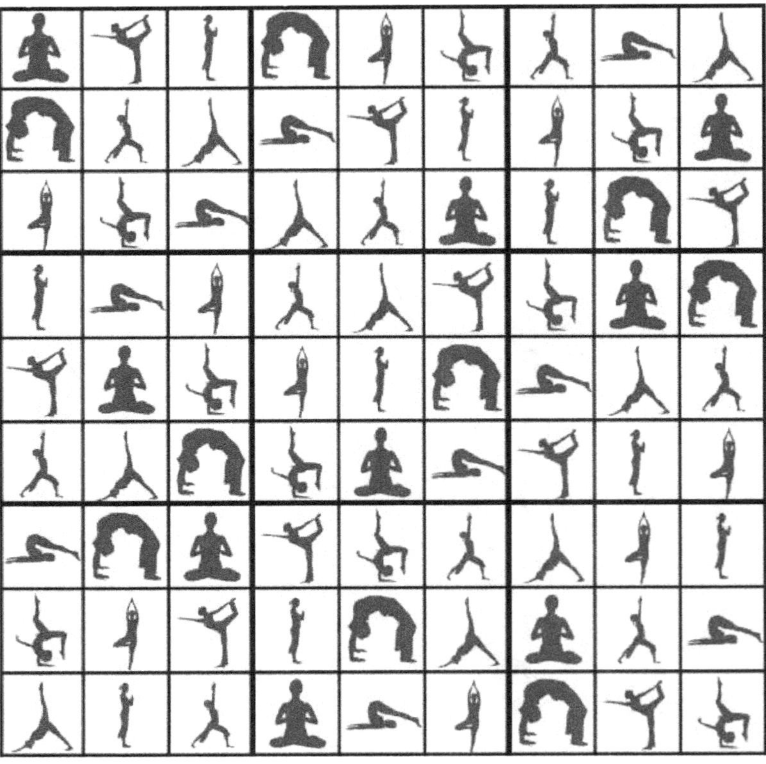

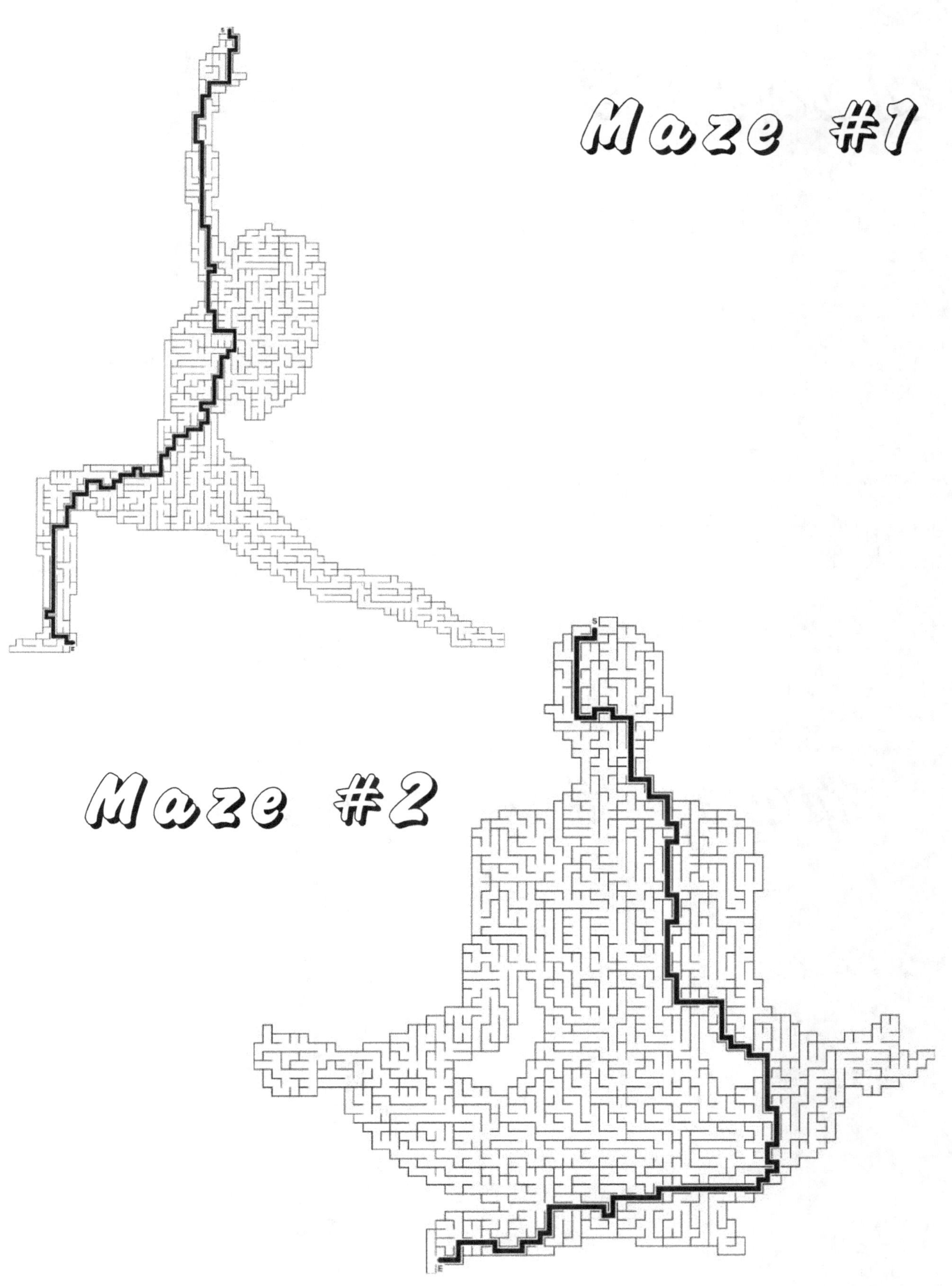

Maze #1
Maze #2

Maze #3

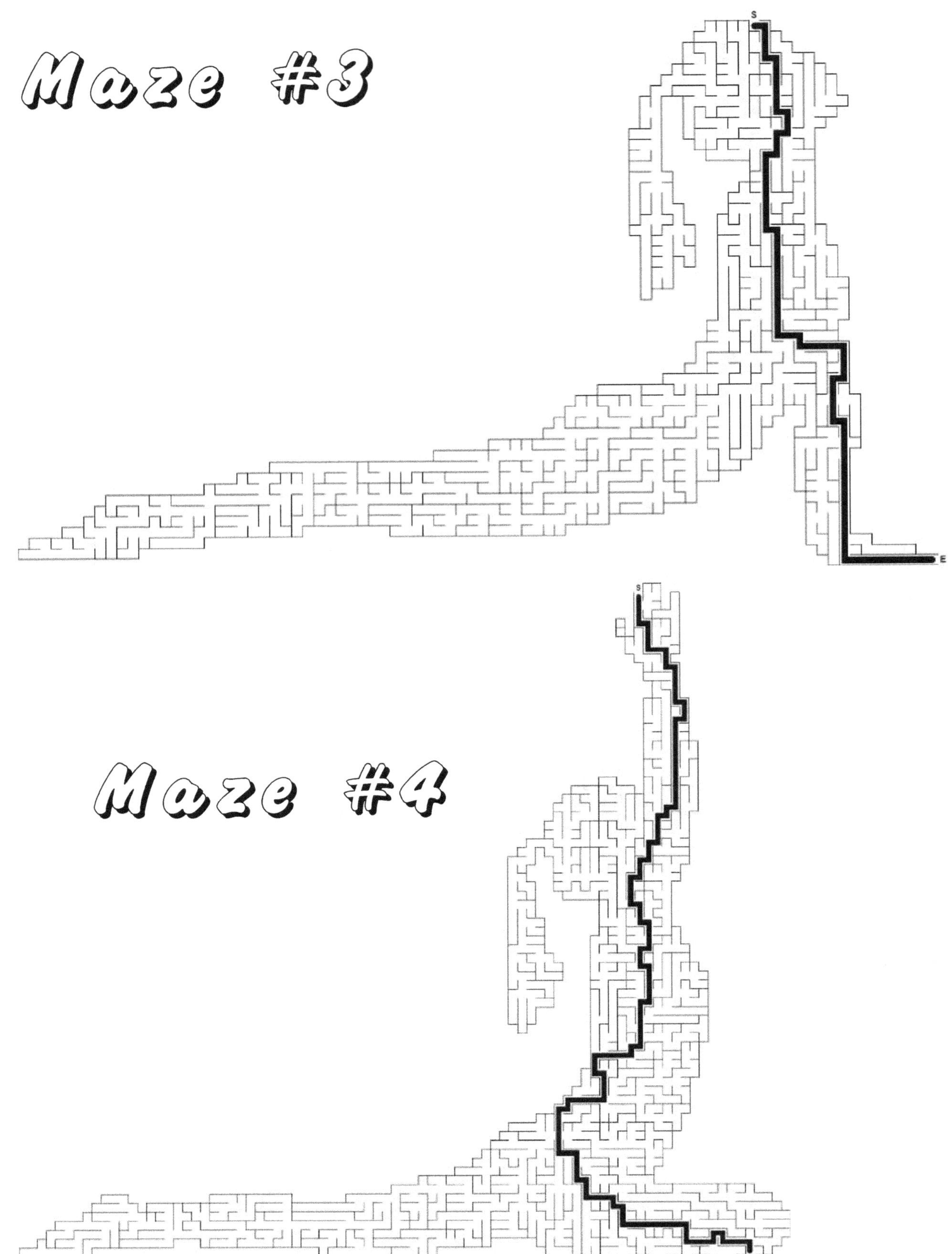

Maze #4

Maze #5

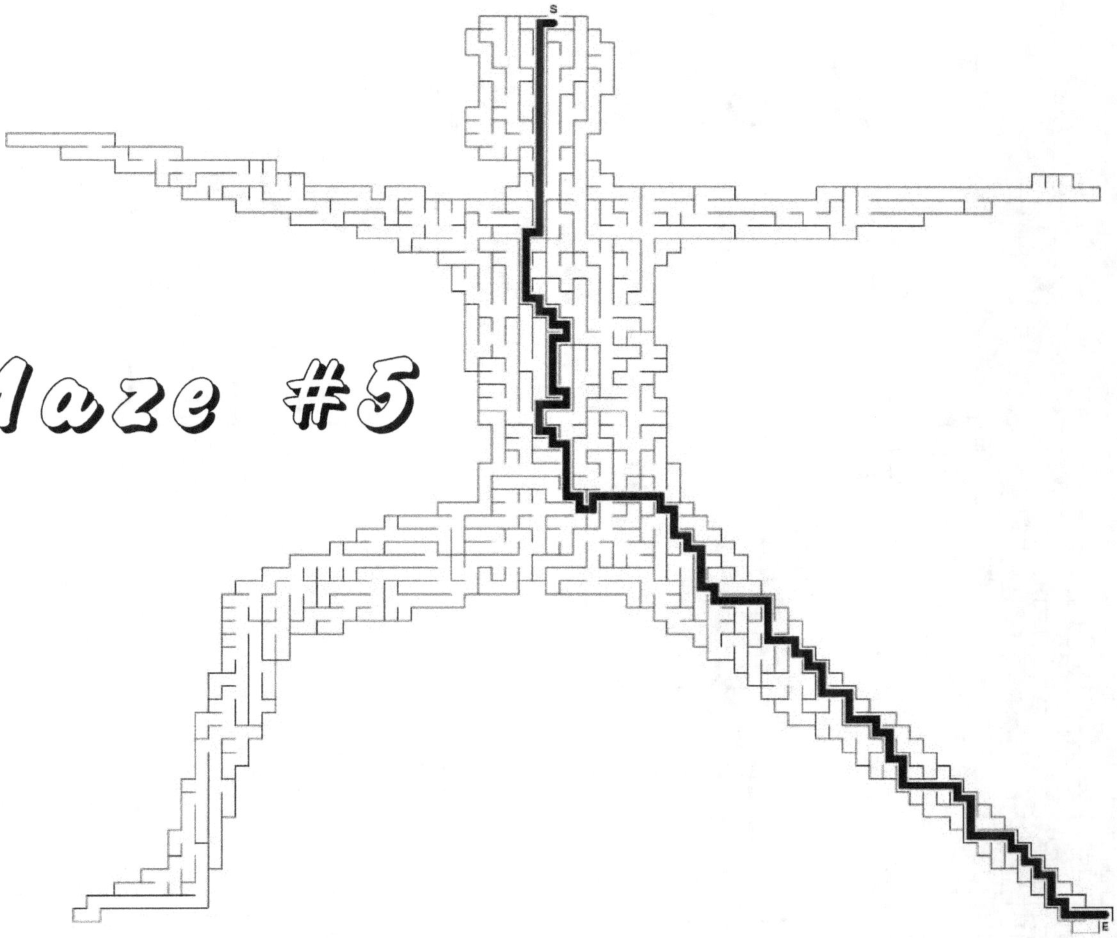

Maze #6

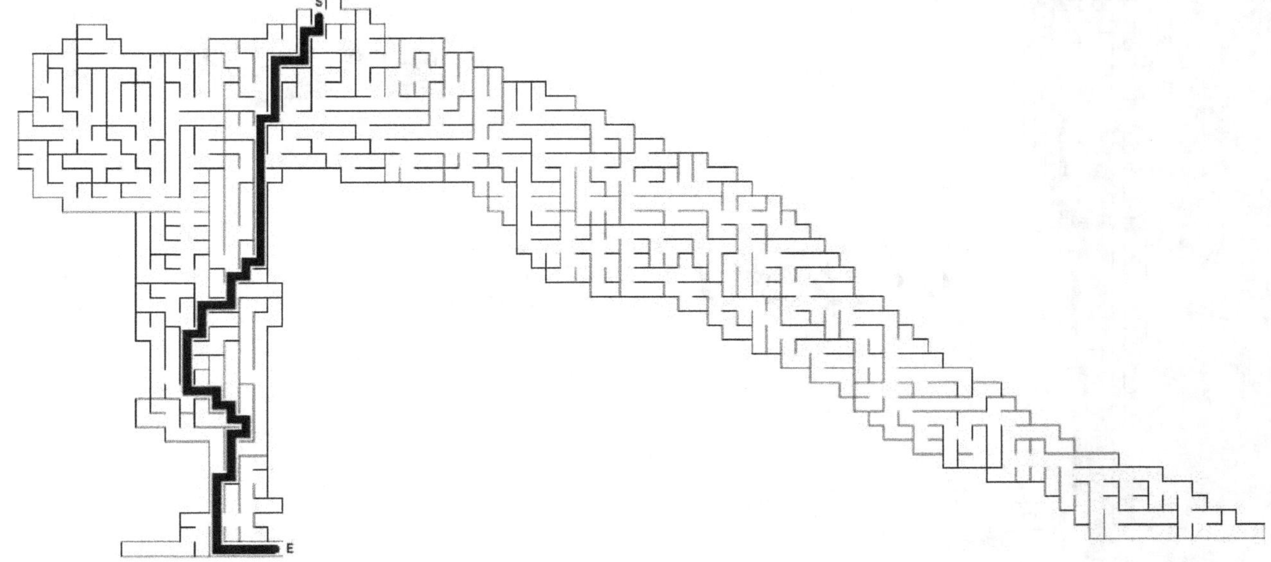

Maze #7

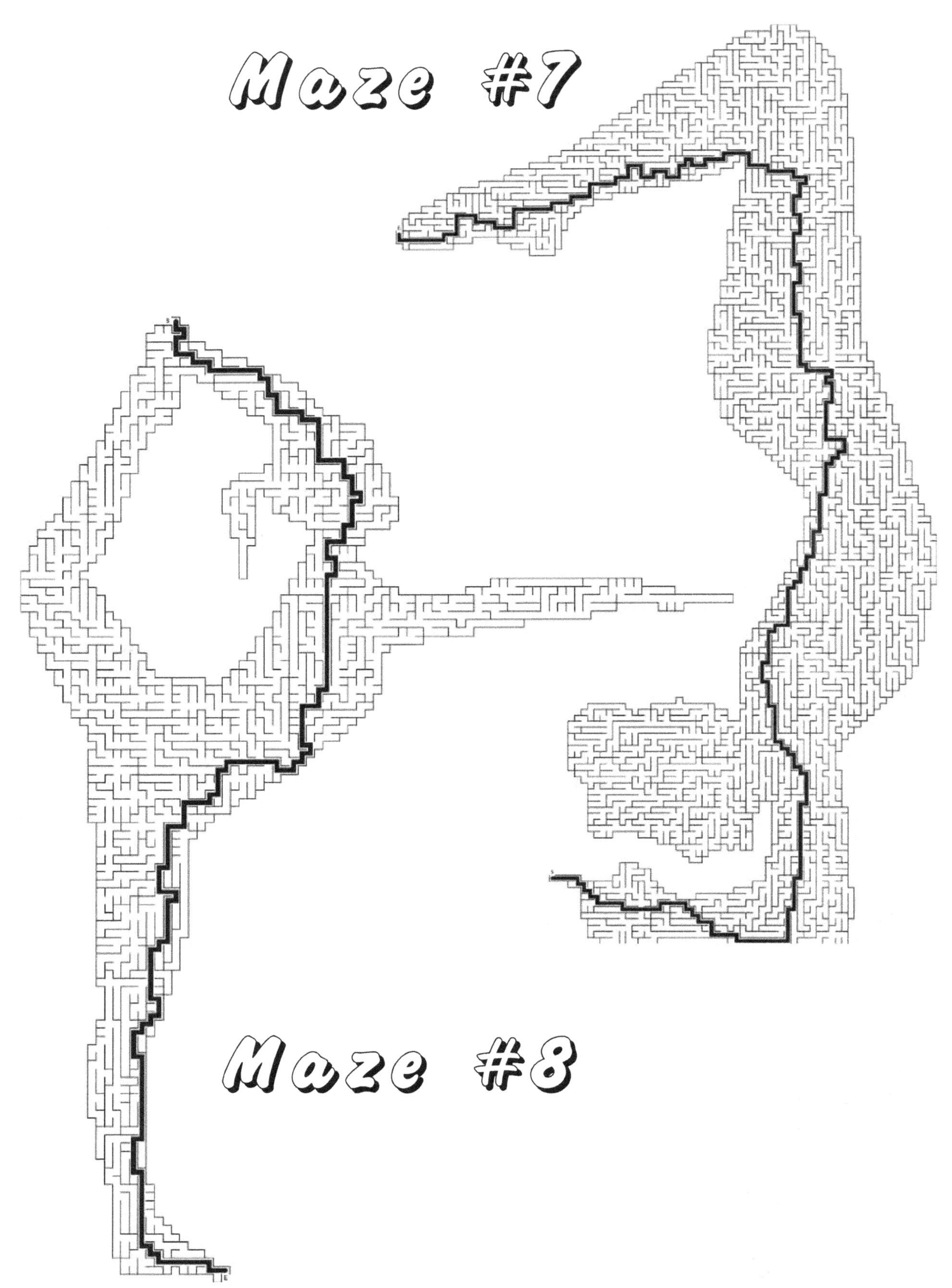

Maze #8

Maze #9

Maze #10

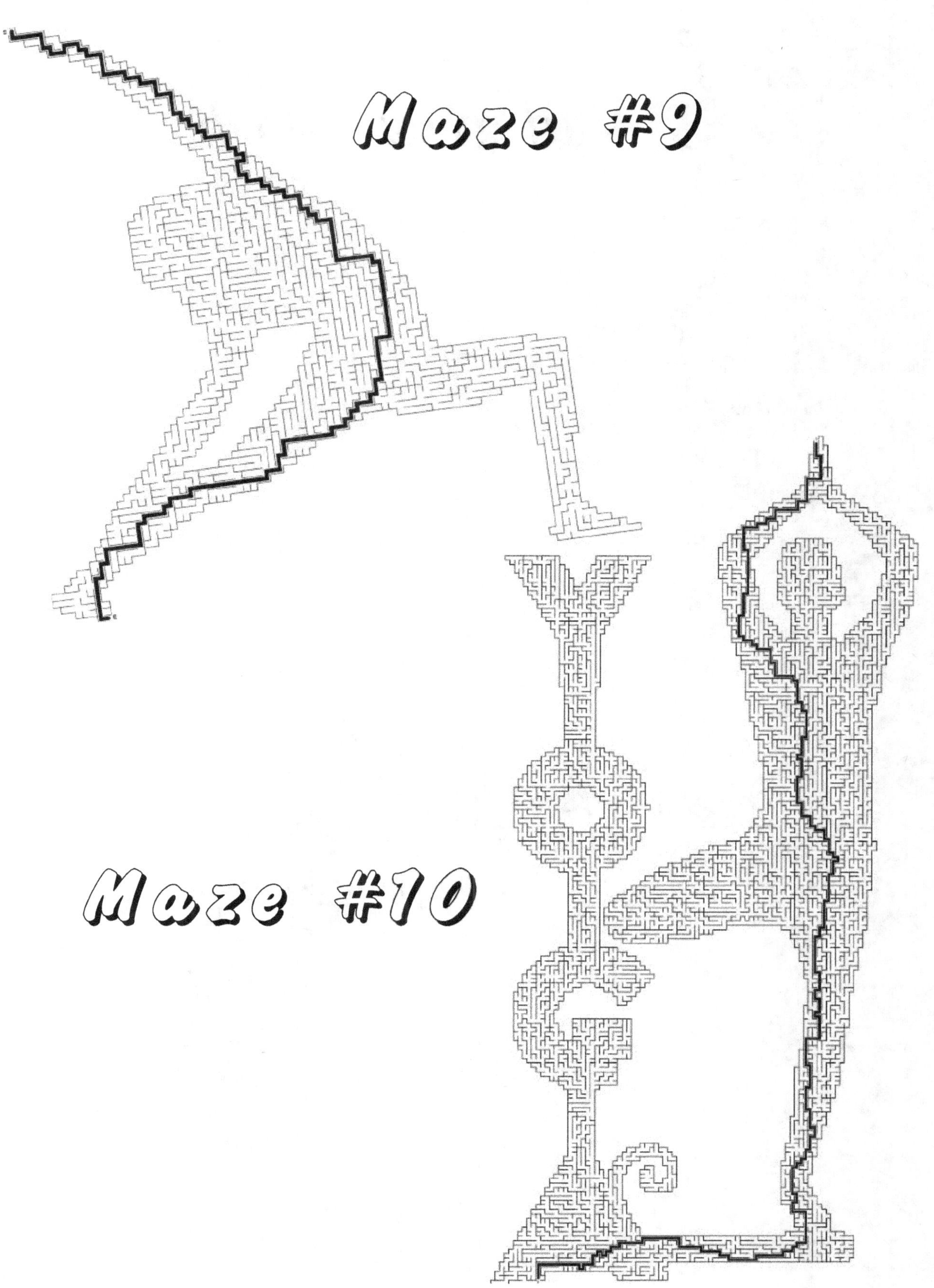

Maze #11

Maze #12

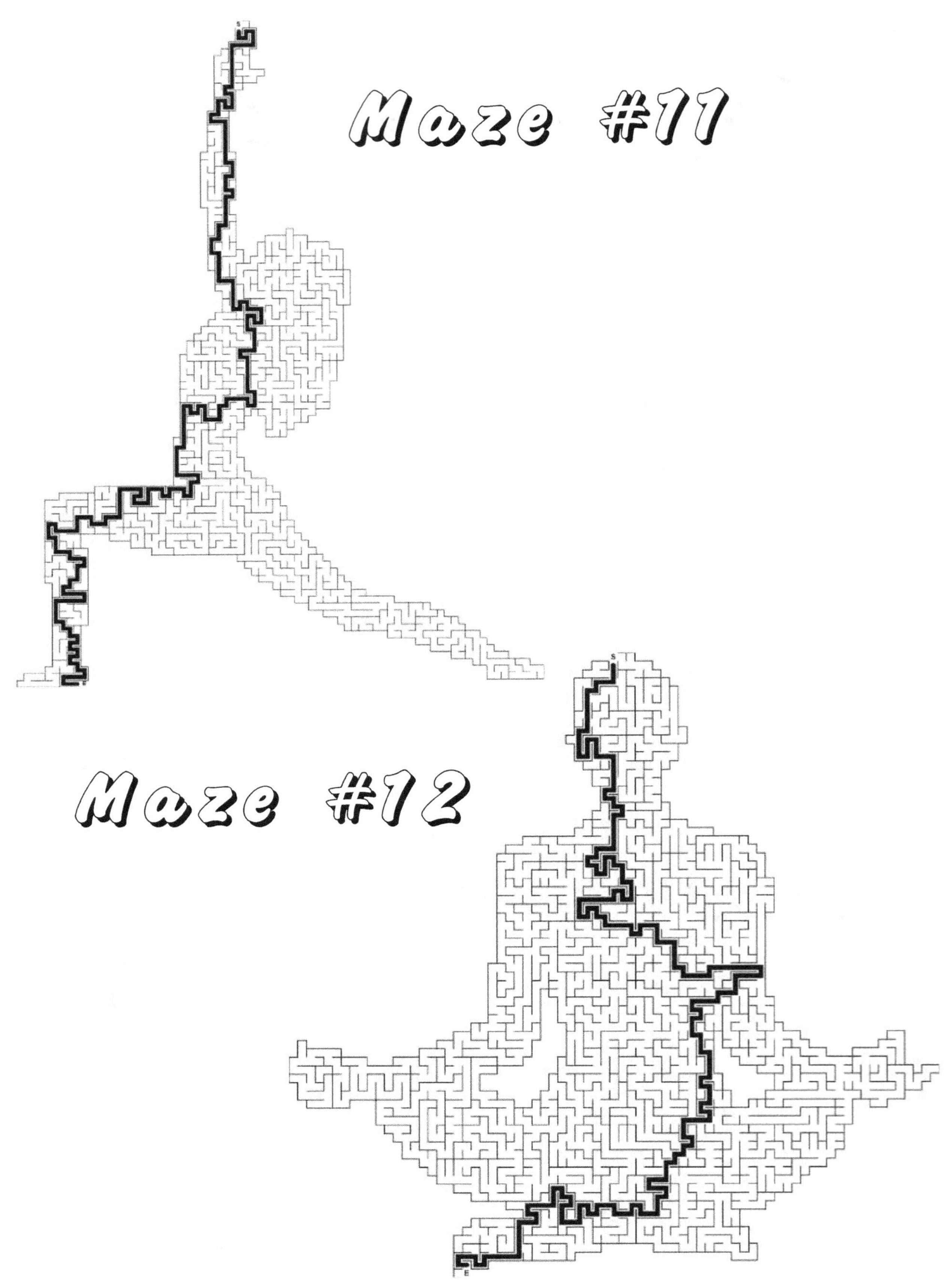

Maze #13

Maze #14

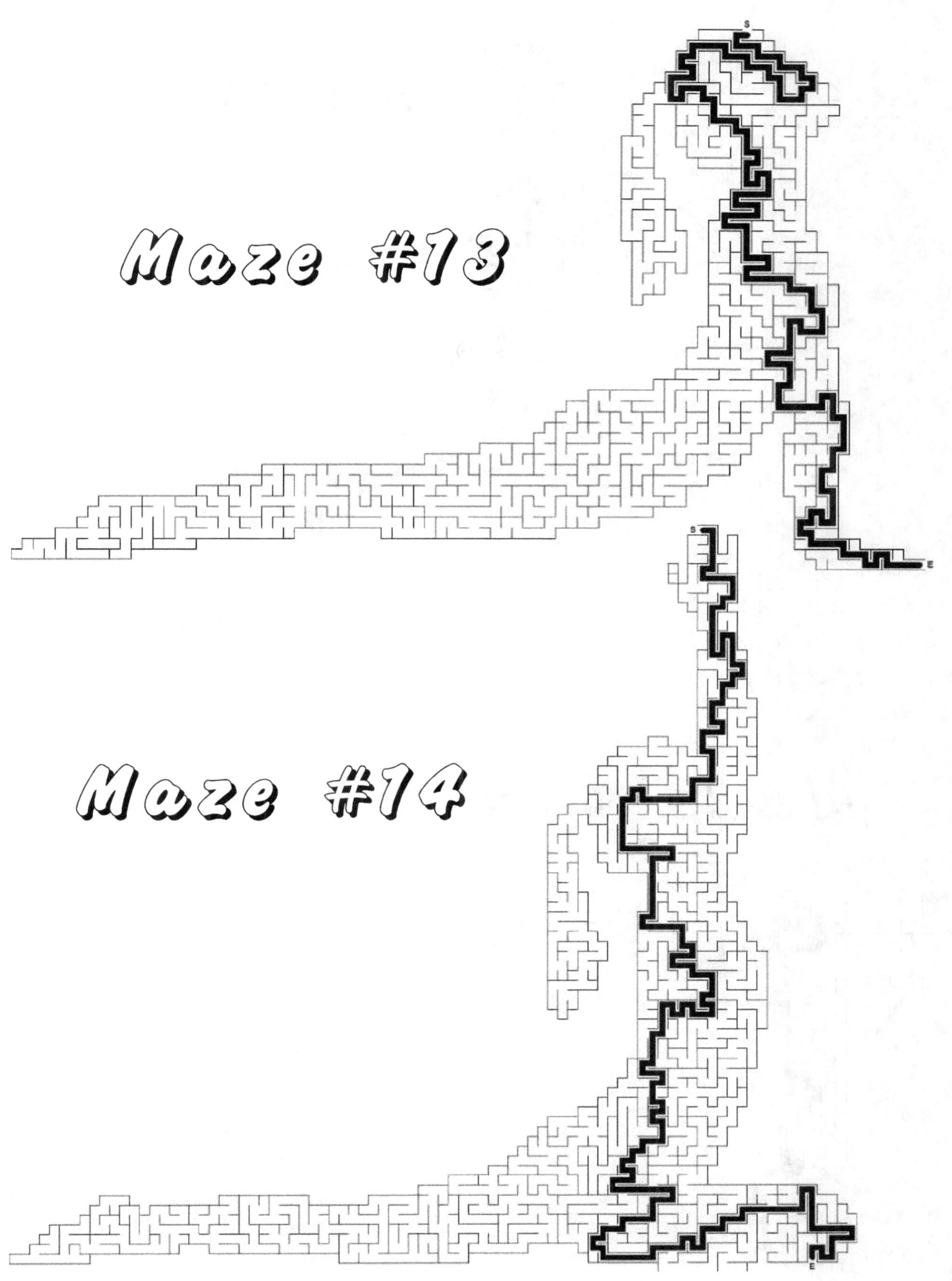

Maze #15

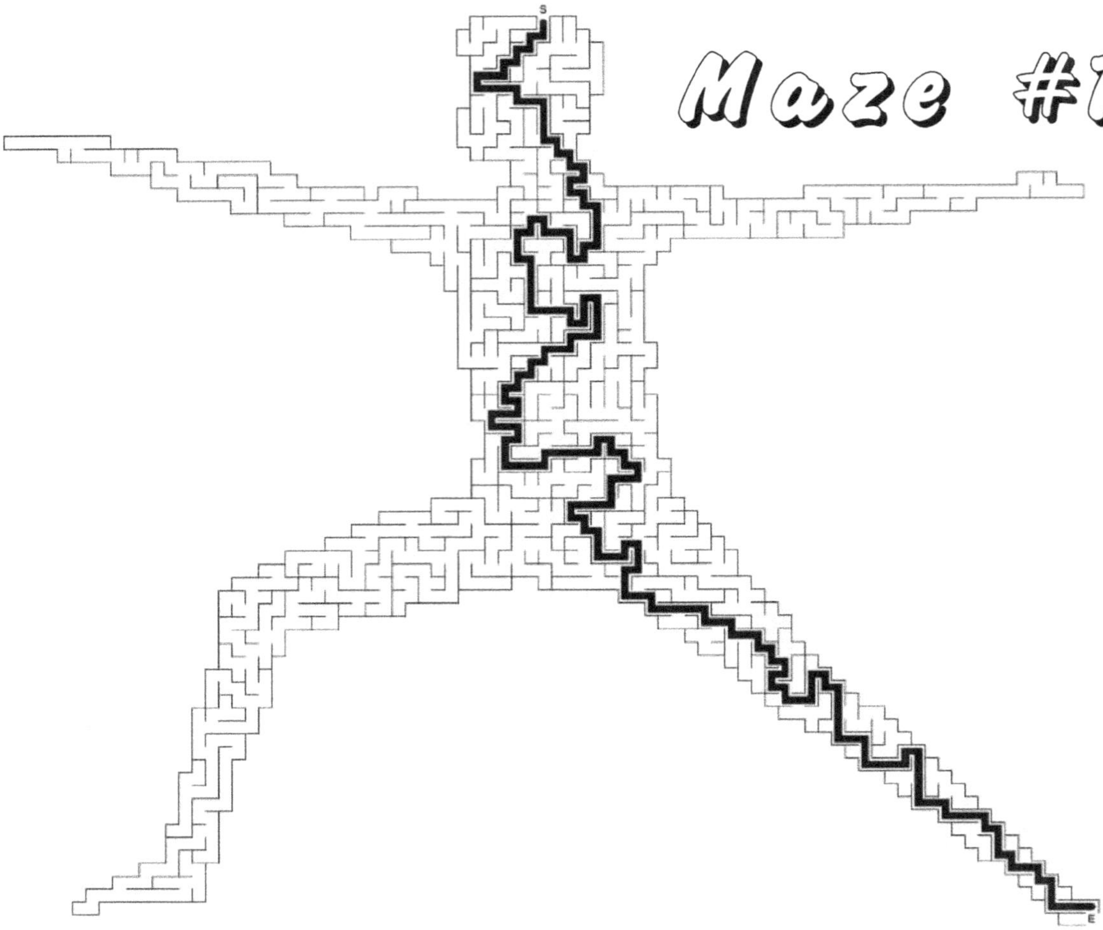

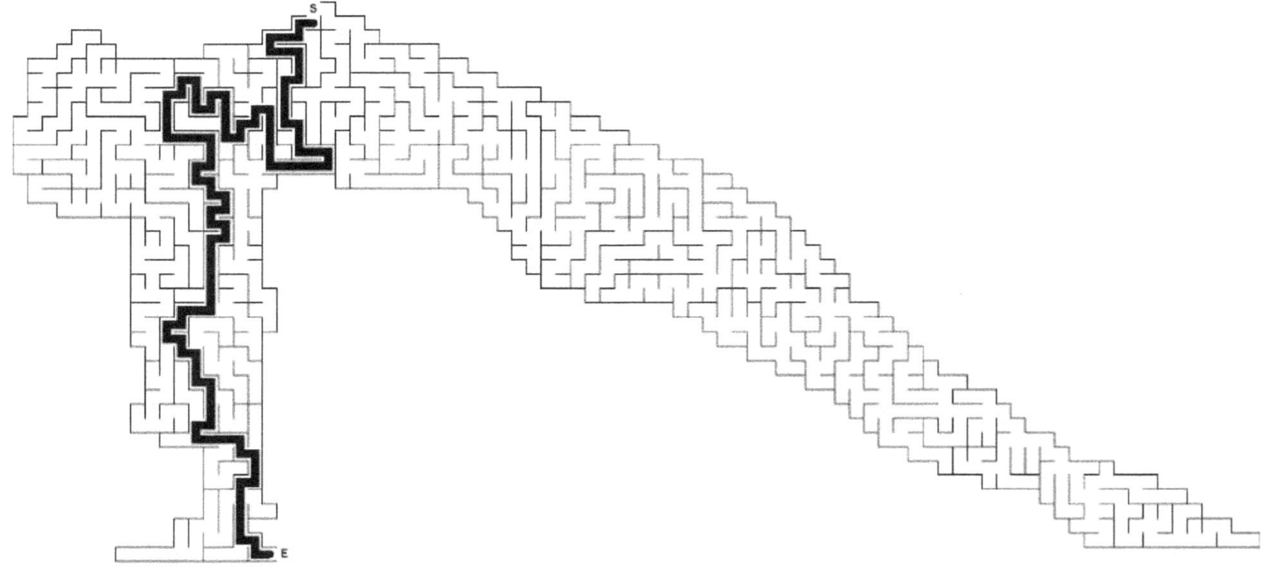

Maze #16

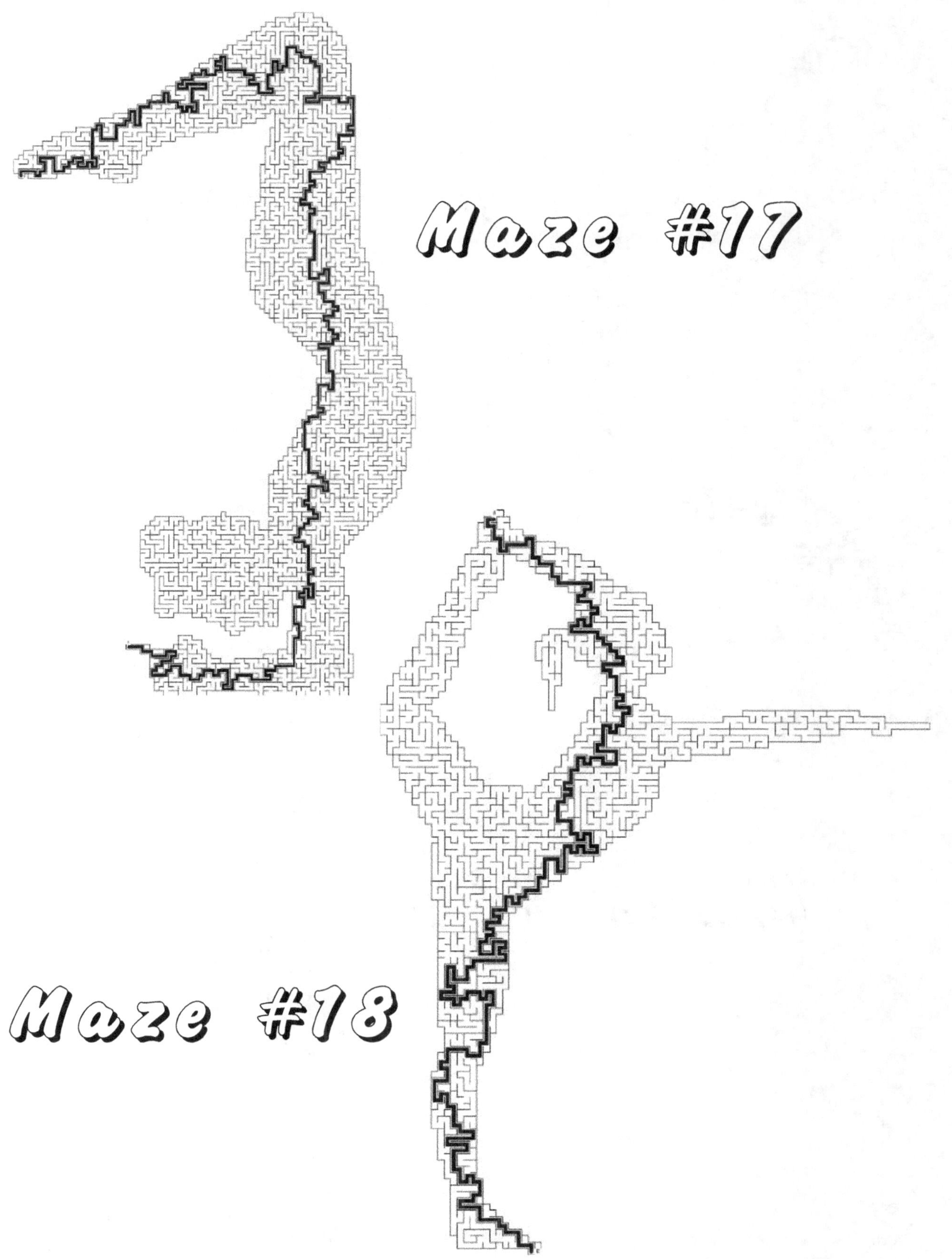

Maze #17
Maze #18

Maze #19

Maze #20

Maze #21

Maze #22

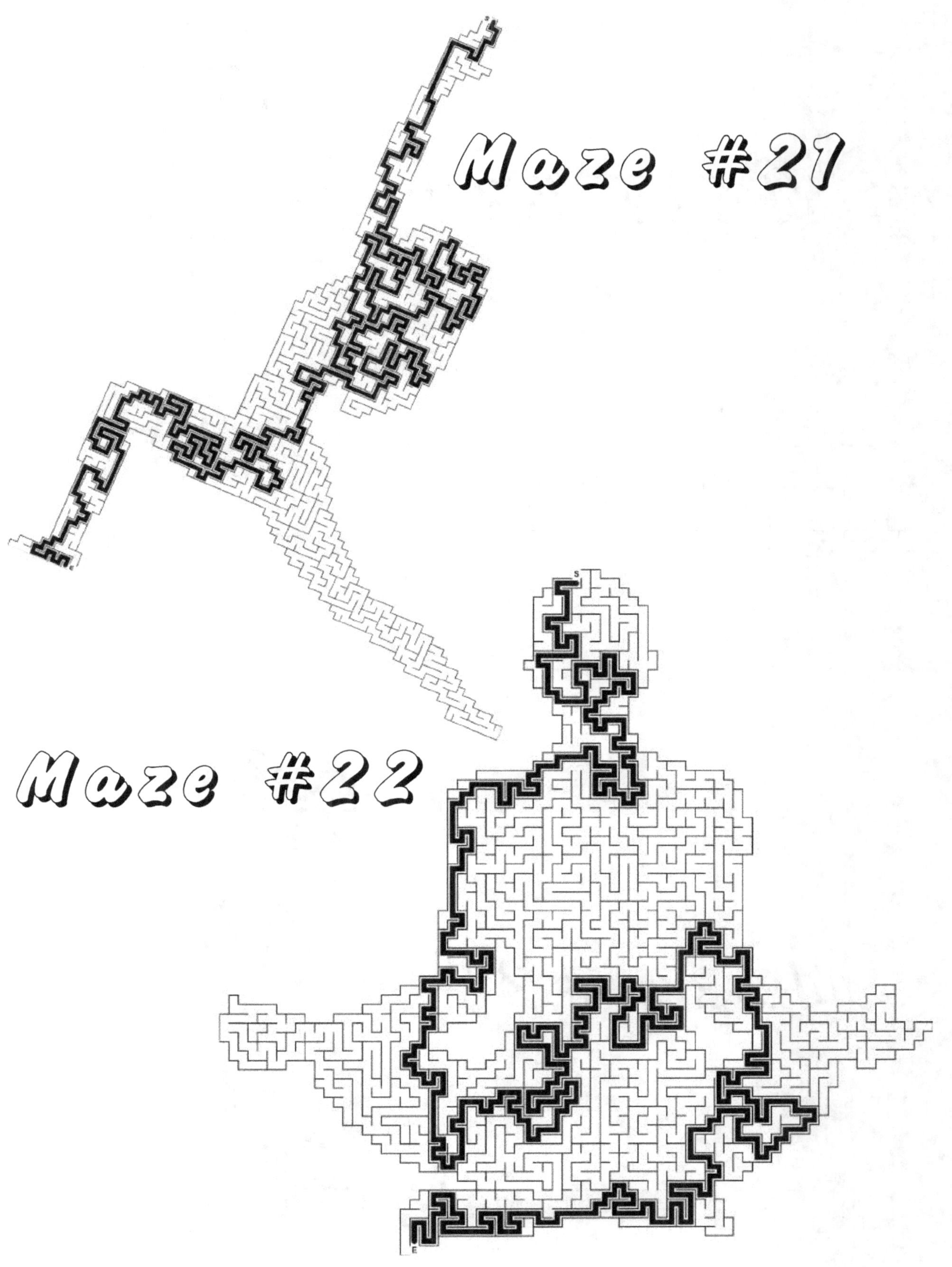

Maze #23

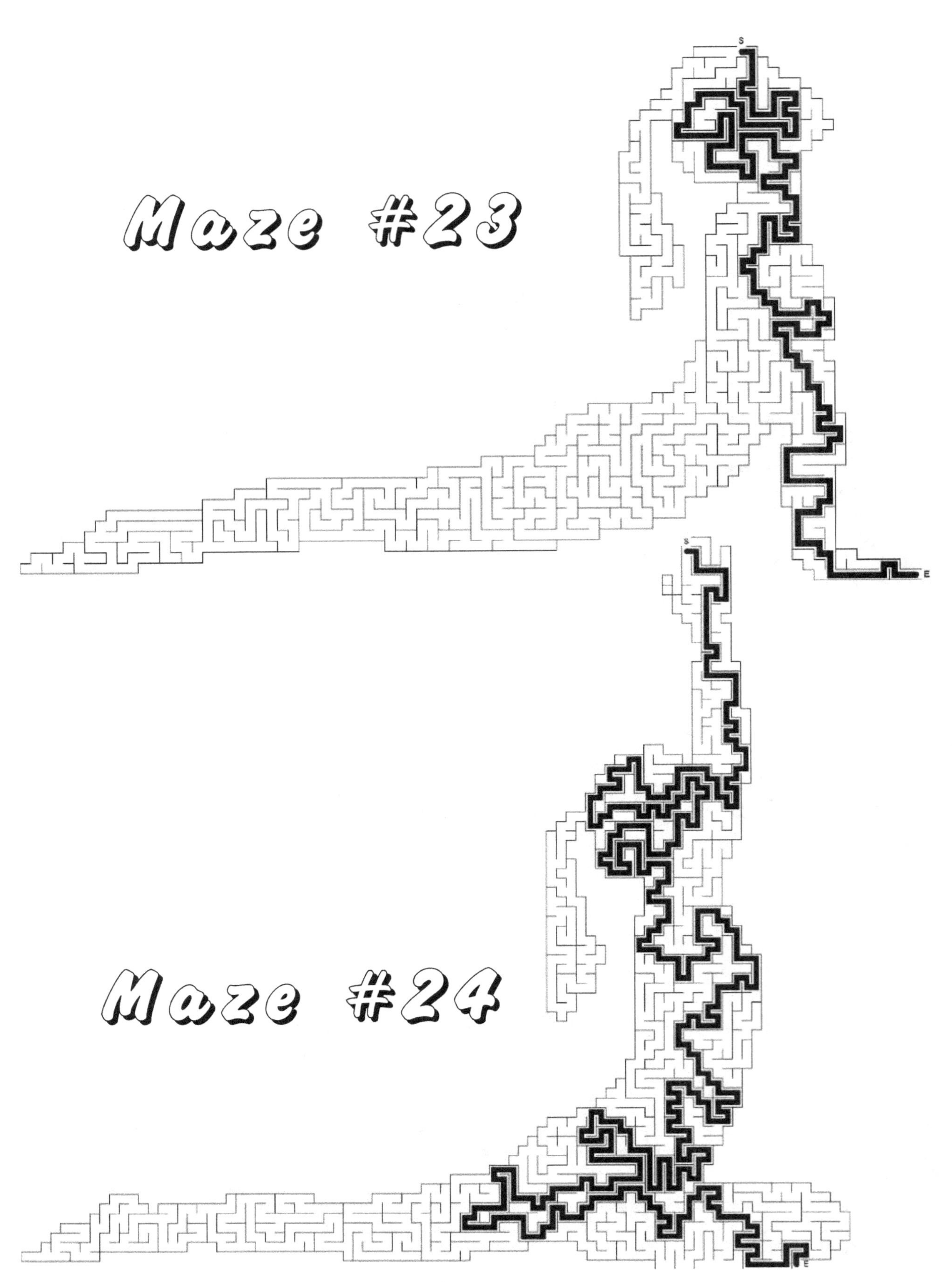

Maze #24

Maze #25

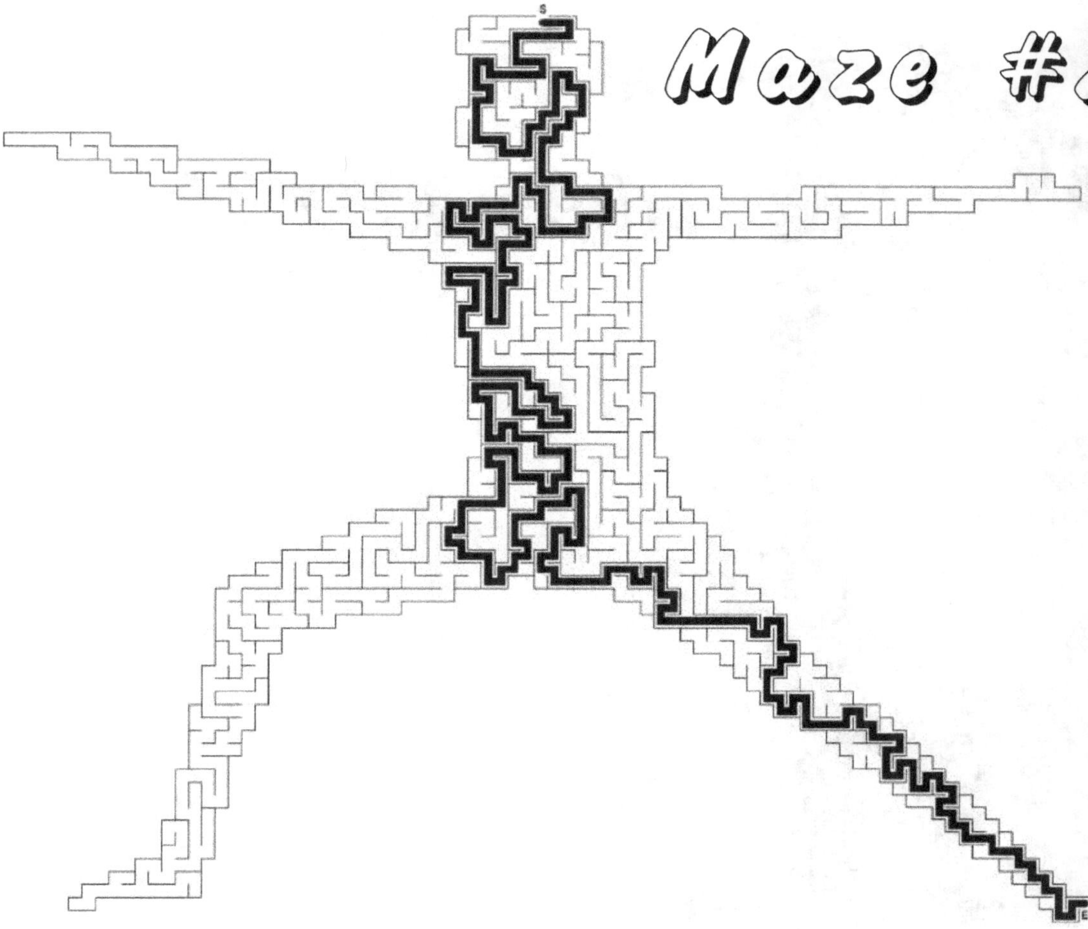

Maze #26

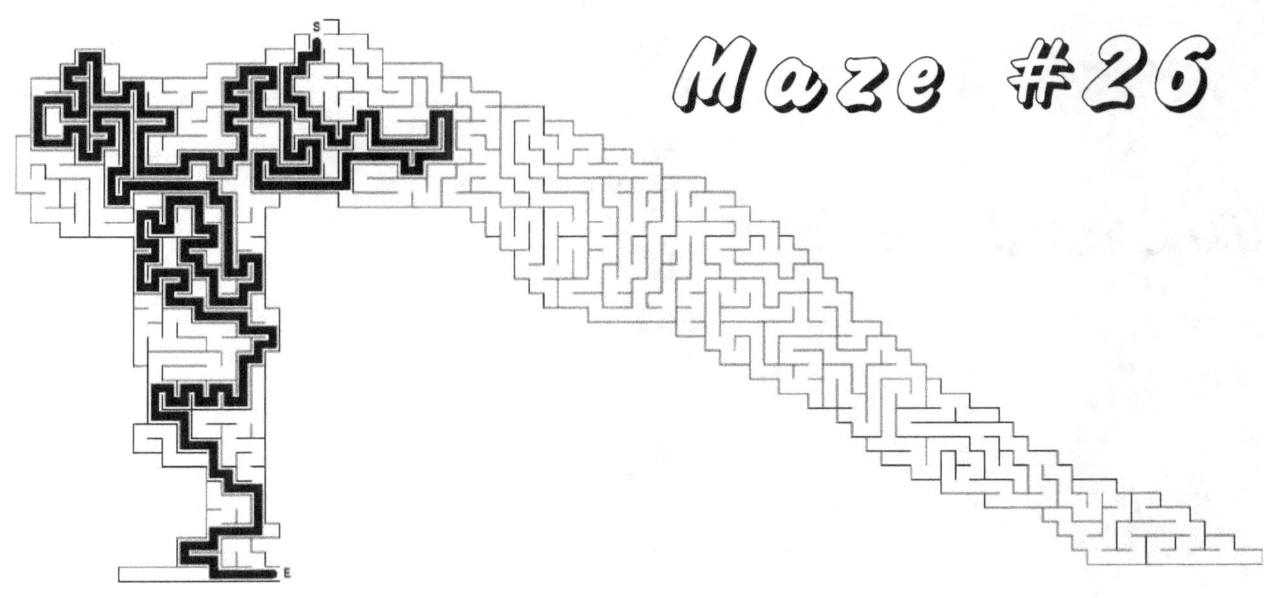

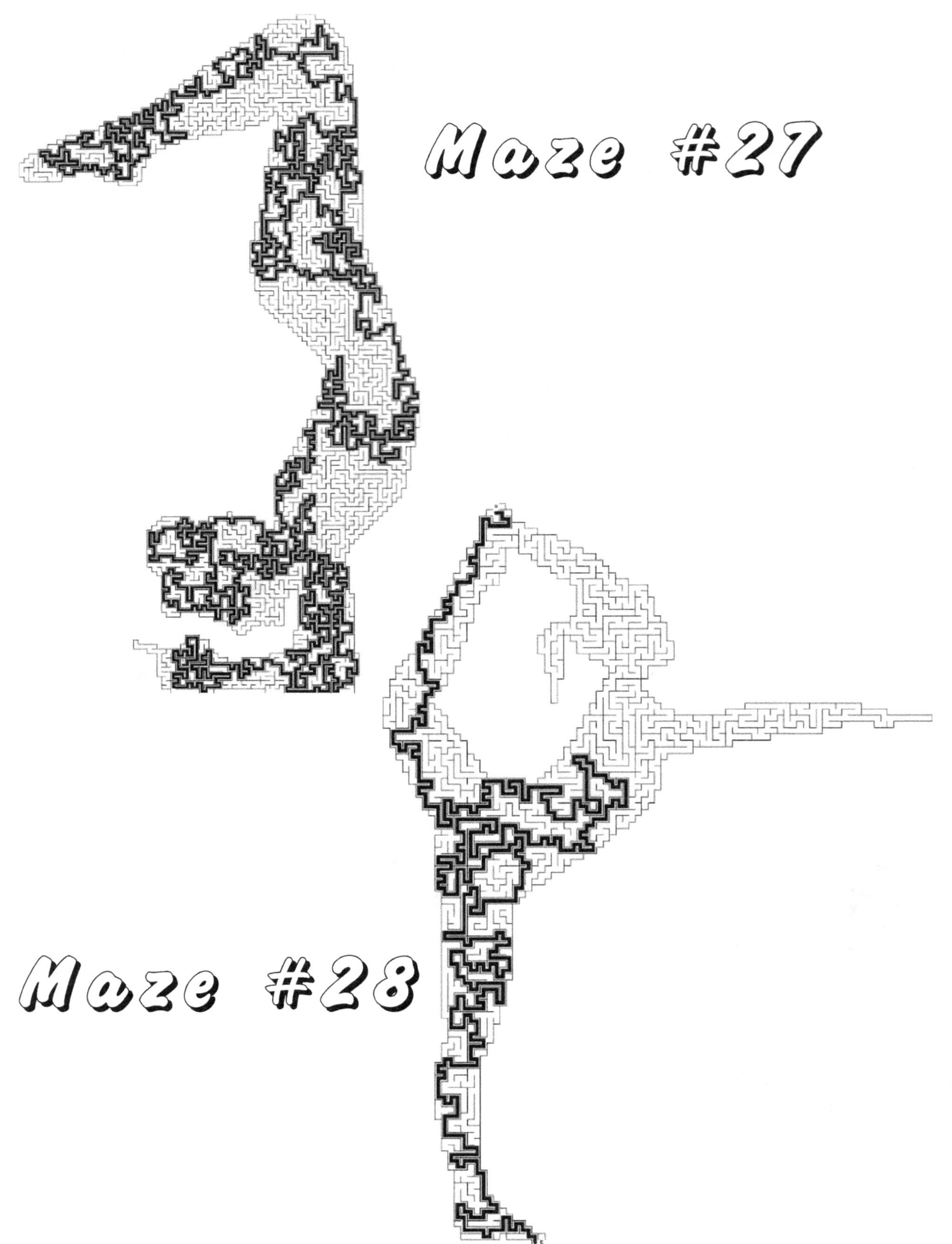

Maze #27
Maze #28

Maze #29

Maze #30

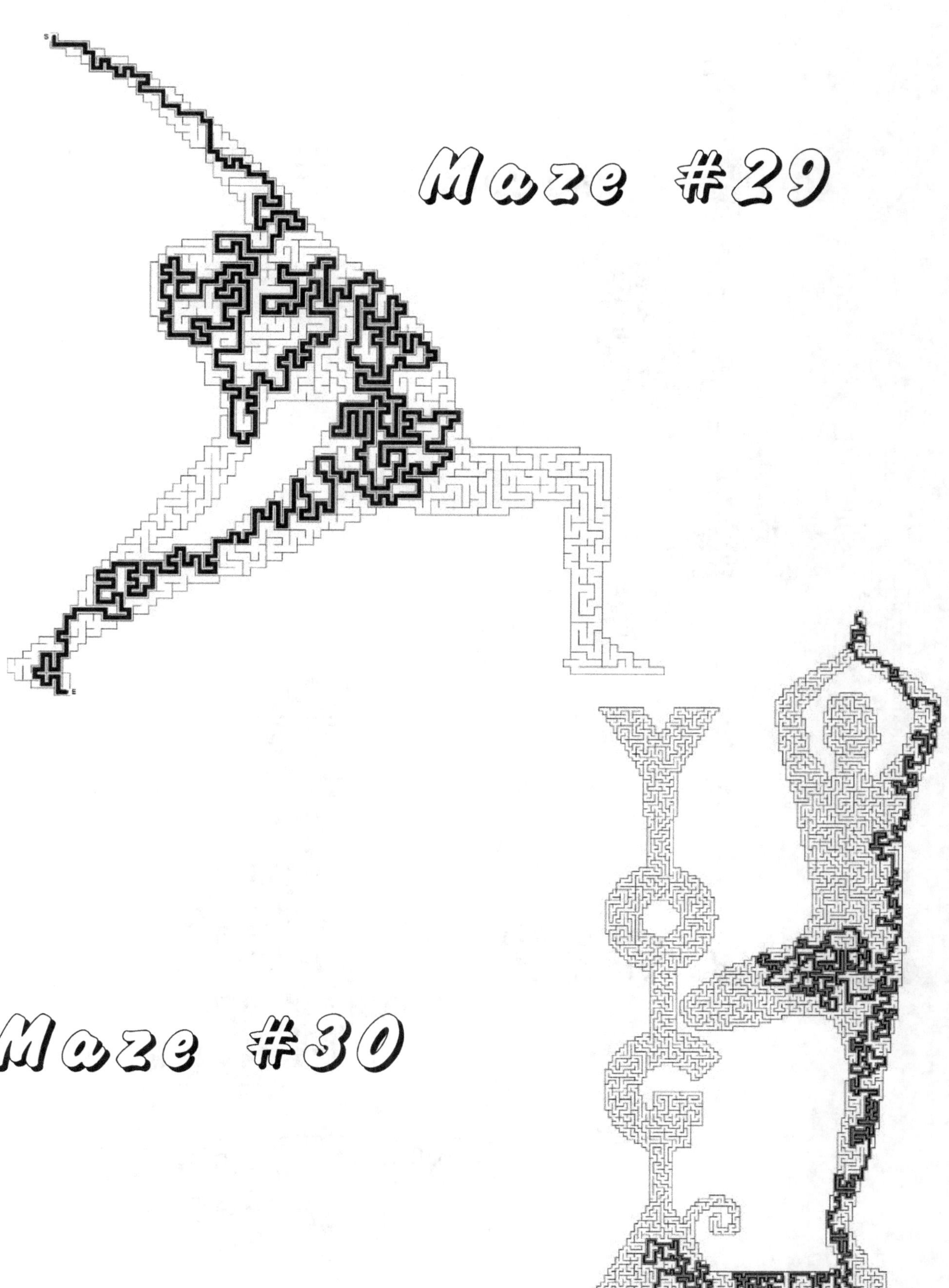

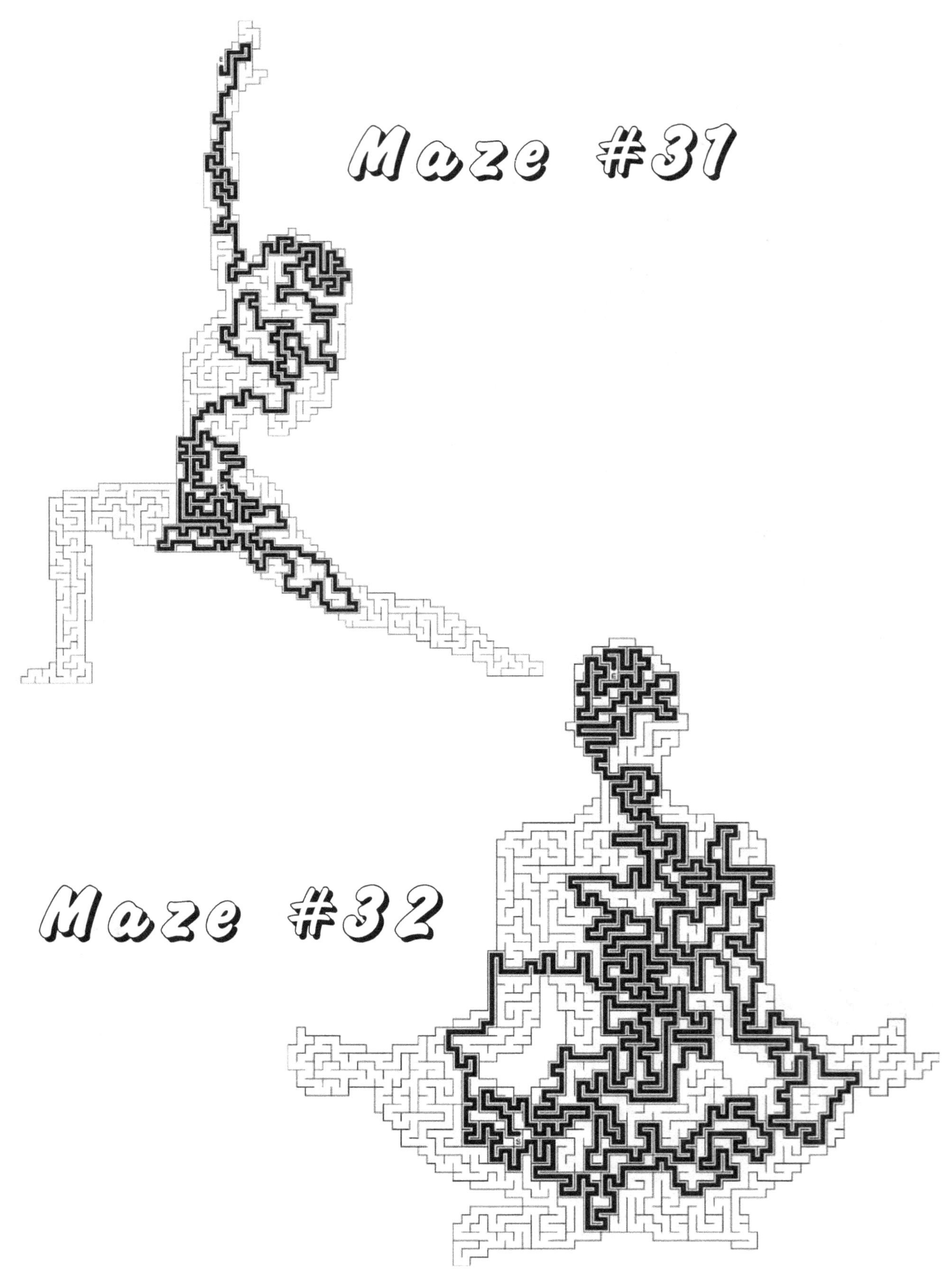
Maze #31
Maze #32

Maze #33

Maze #34

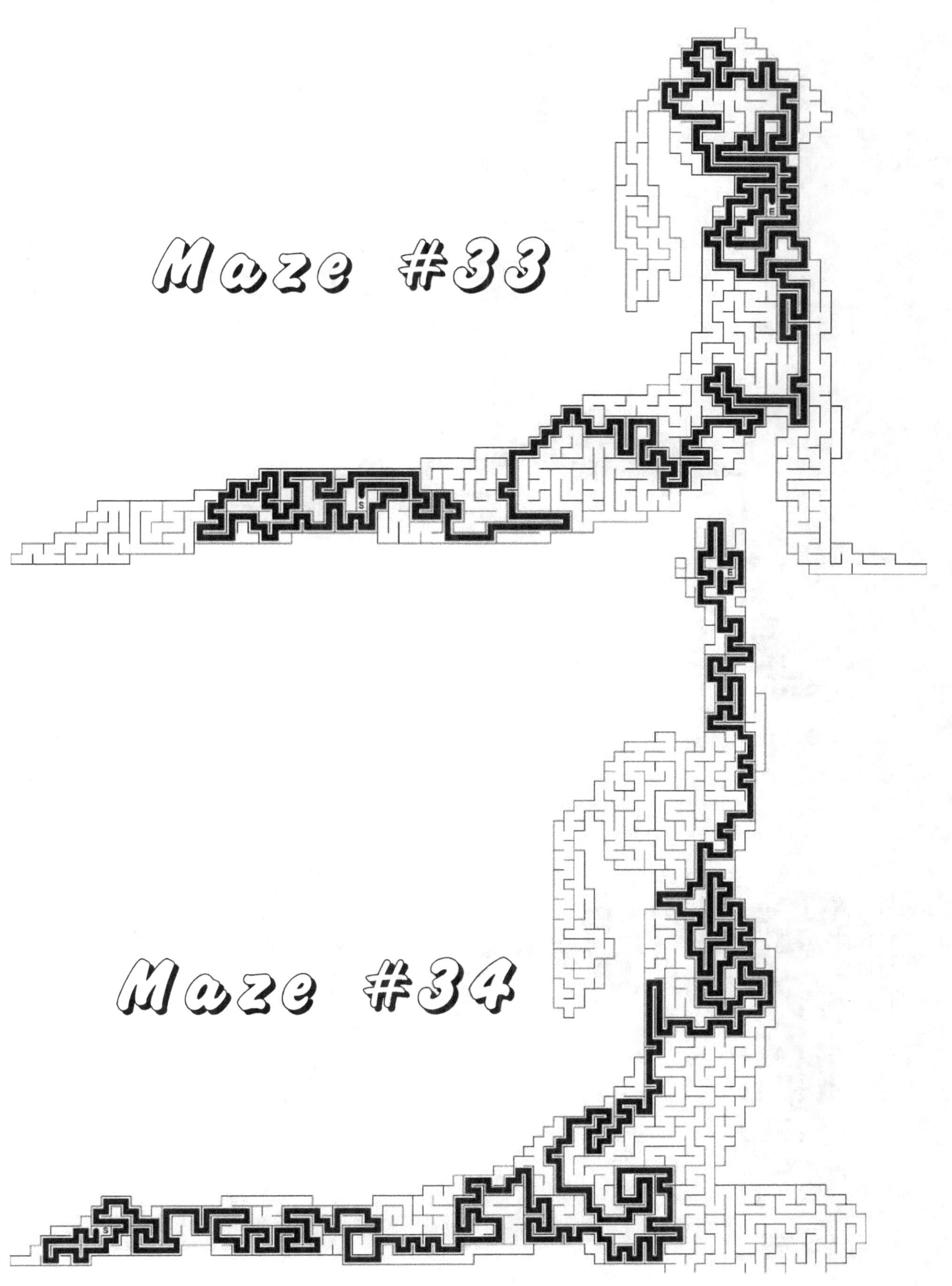

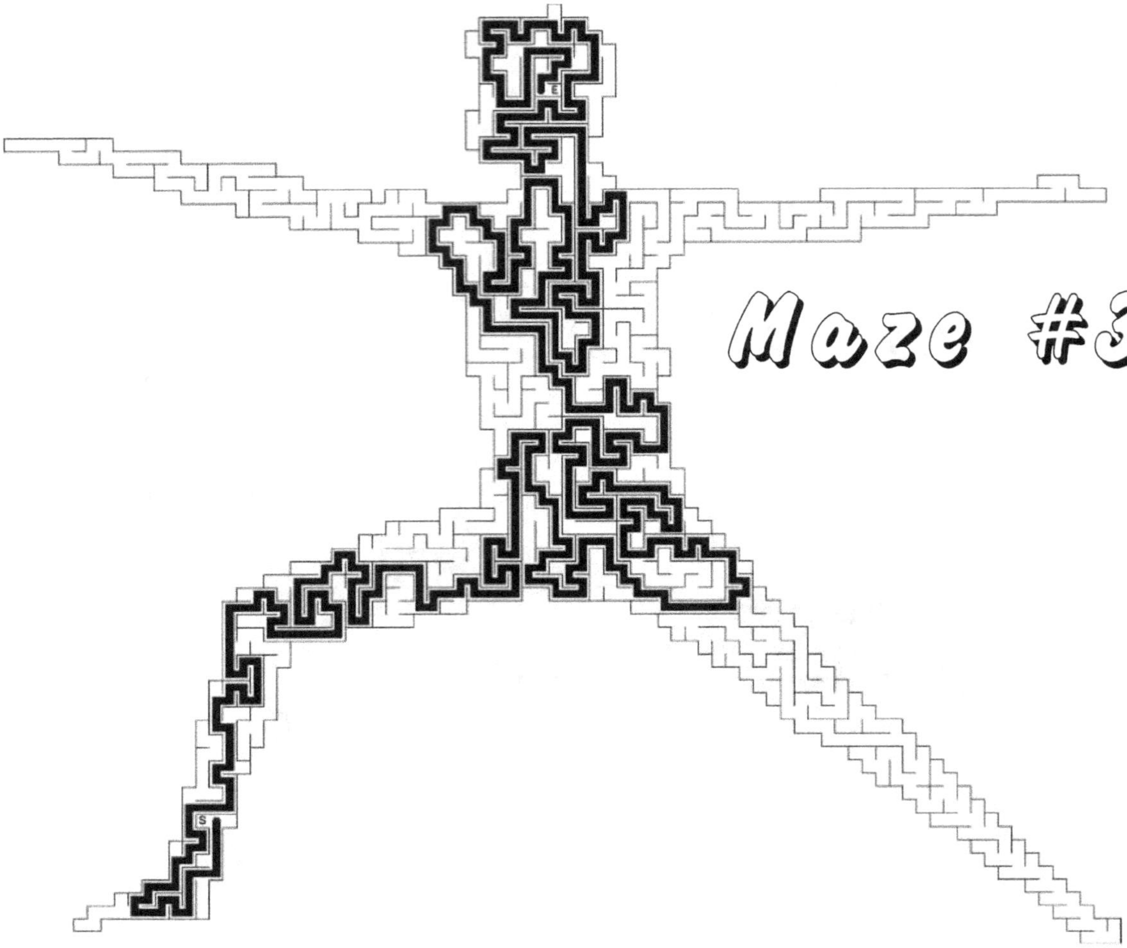

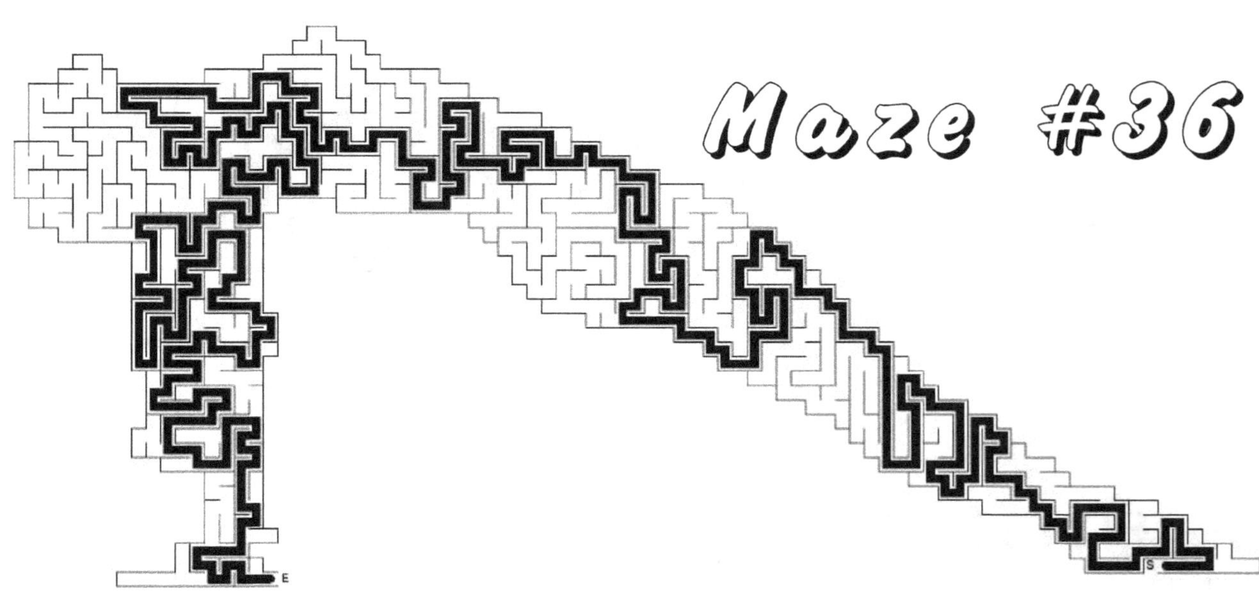

Maze #35

Maze #36

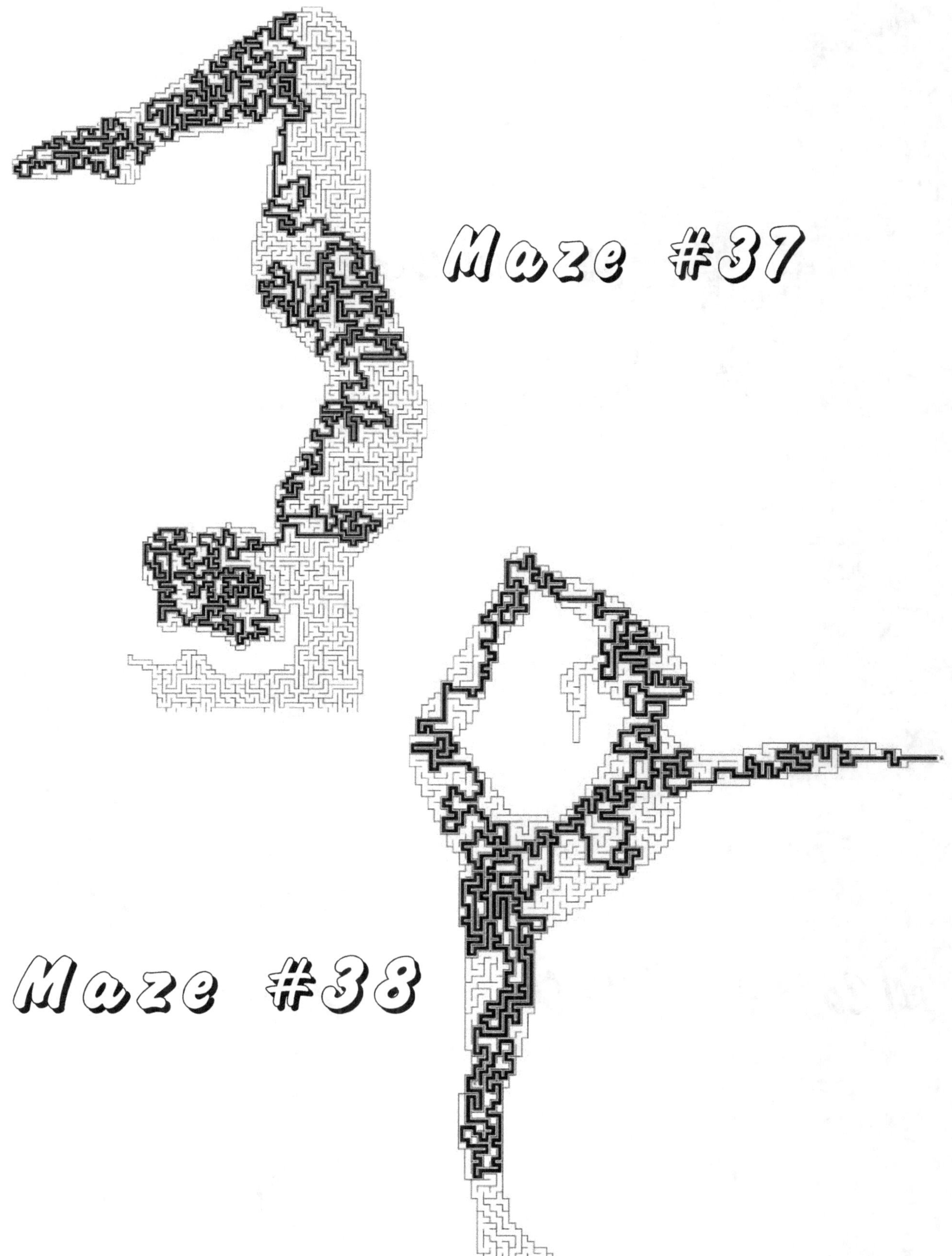

Maze #37
Maze #38

Maze #39

Maze #40

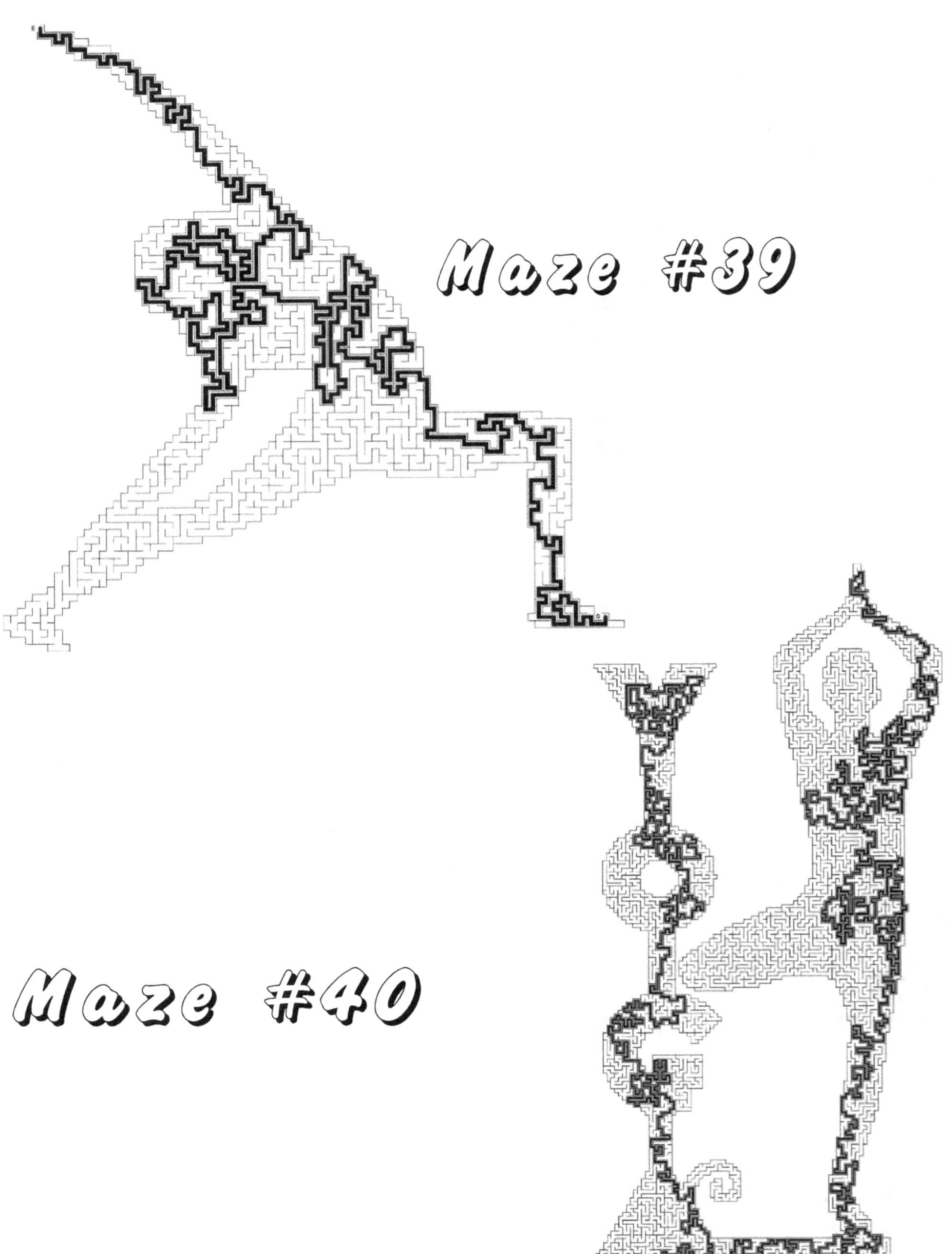

Want Even MORE Themed Puzzle fun?
Try These!

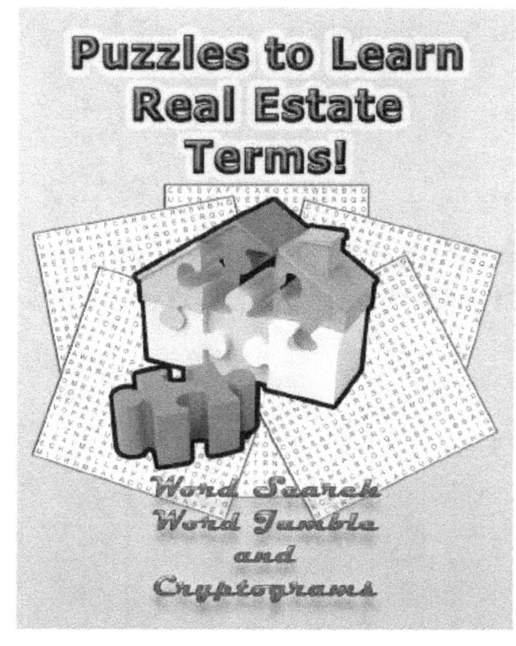

Puzzles To Learn Real Estate Terms!
https://www.amazon.com/dp/1079170758

Music Themed Puzzles
https://www.amazon.com/dp/B07Y4LM6NZ

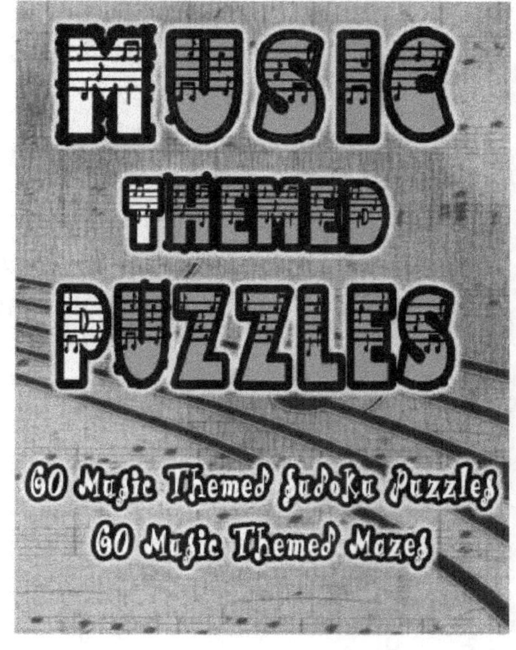

Want Even MORE Themed Puzzle fun?
Try These!

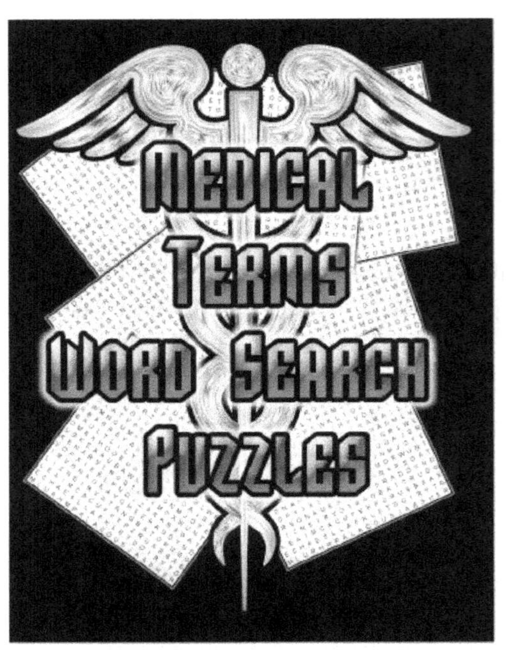

Medical Terms Word Search Puzzles
https://www.amazon.com/dp/1070711772

140 Photography Puzzles
https://www.amazon.com/dp/1070835072

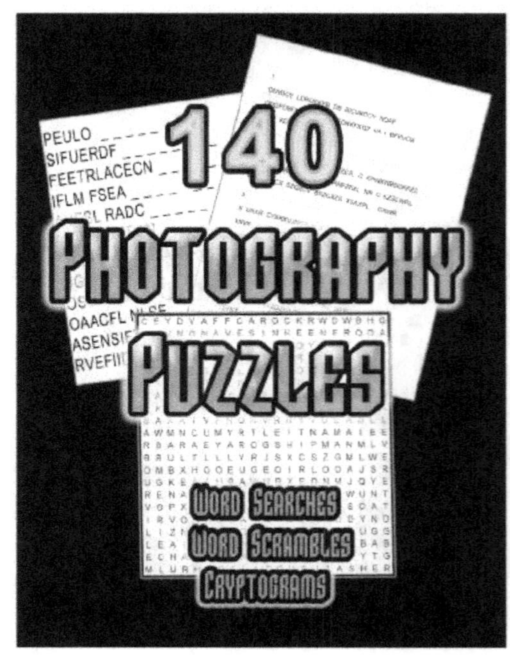

Want Even MORE Themed Puzzle fun?
Try These!

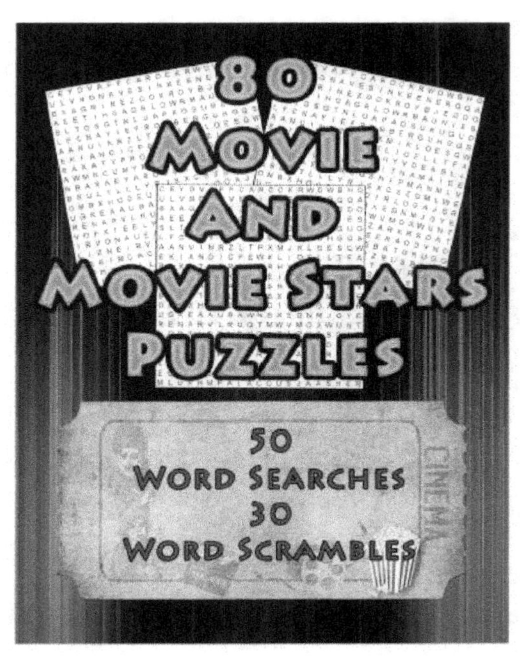

80 Movie And Movie Stars Puzzles
https://www.amazon.com/dp/1071448099

Music's Greatest Hits
100 Word Search Puzzles
https://www.amazon.com/dp/107233397X

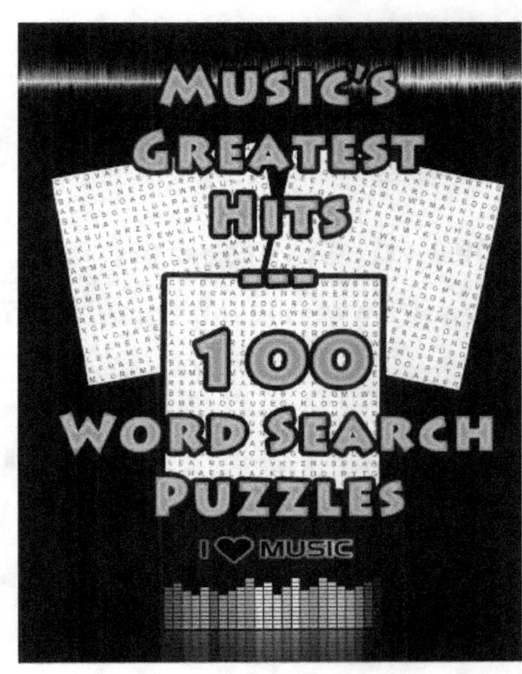

Want Even MORE Themed Puzzle fun?
Try These!

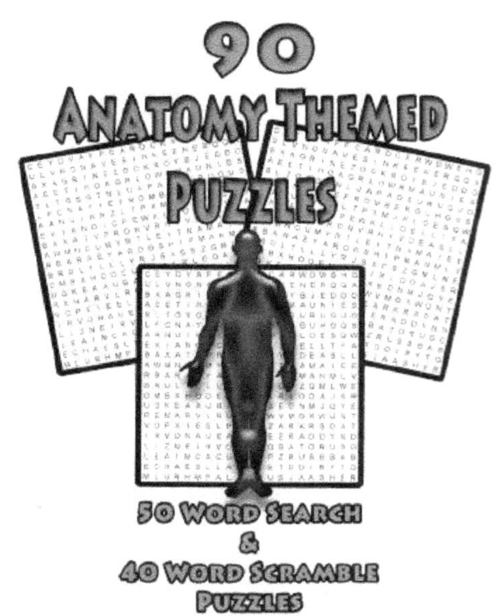

90 Anatomy Themed Puzzles
https://www.amazon.com/dp/1072719177

300 LOL Cryptograms

https://www.amazon.com/dp/107597934X

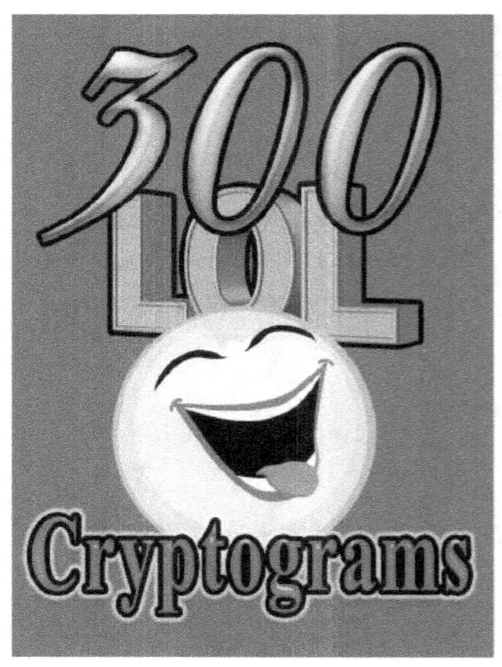

Want Even MORE Puzzle fun?
Try These Holiday Themed Puzzles!

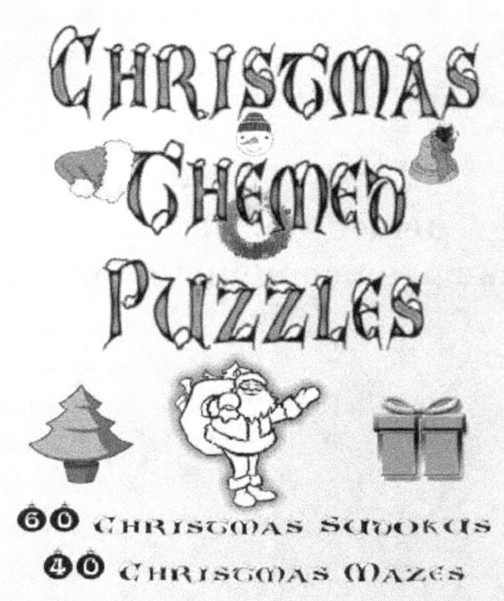

Christmas Themed Puzzles
https://www.amazon.com/dp/1693275082

Halloween Themed Puzzles
https://www.amazon.com/dp/169285724X

Want Even MORE Puzzle fun?
Try These Holiday Themed Puzzles!

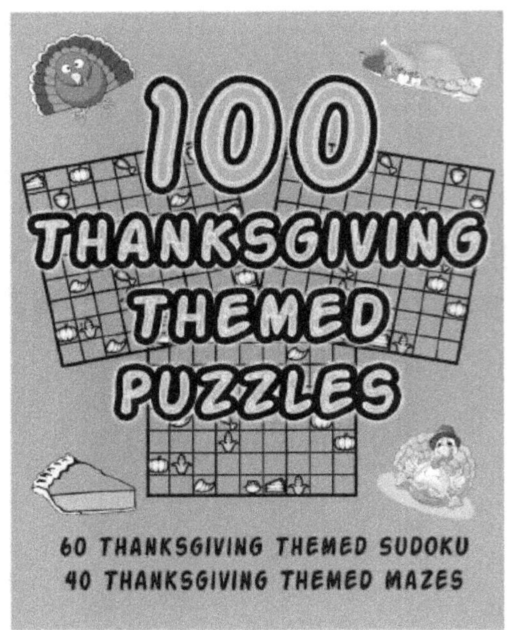

Thanksgiving Themed Puzzles
https://www.amazon.com/dp/1695000056

New Year Themed Puzzles
https://www.amazon.com/dp/169568043X

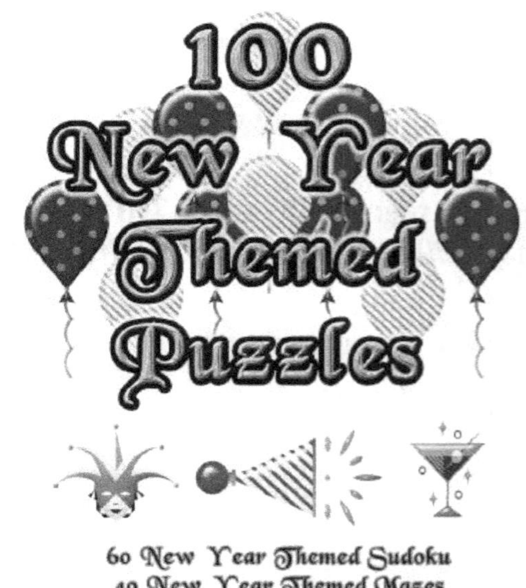

Want Even MORE Puzzle fun?
Try These Holiday Themed Puzzles!

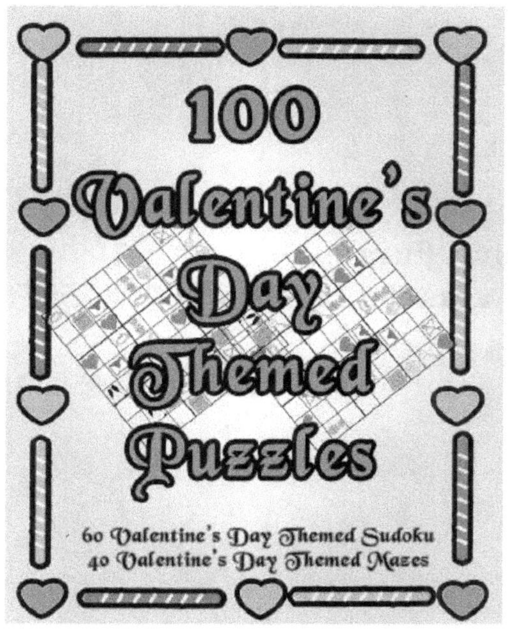

Valentine's Day Themed Puzzles
https://www.amazon.com/dp/1696425603

St. Patrick's Day Themed Puzzles
https://www.amazon.com/dp/1697214150

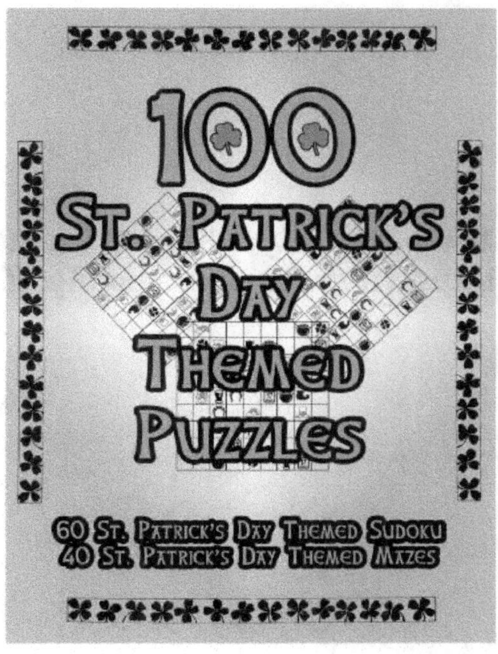

Want Even MORE Puzzle fun?
Try These Holiday Themed Puzzles!

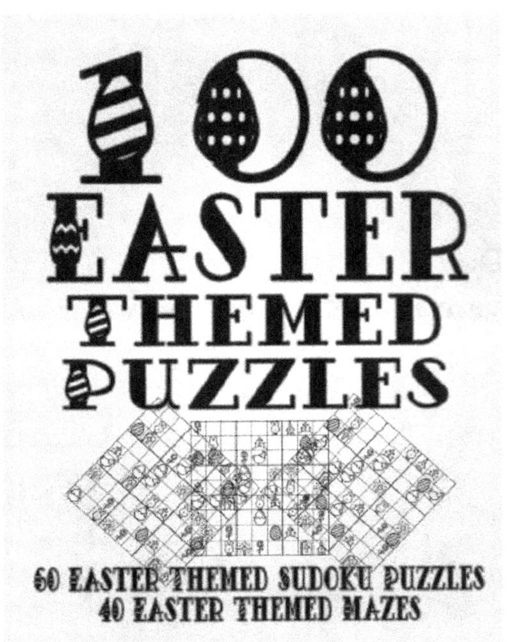

Easter Themed Puzzles
https://www.amazon.com/dp/1697875556

Mother's Day Themed Puzzles
https://www.amazon.com/dp/1698375387

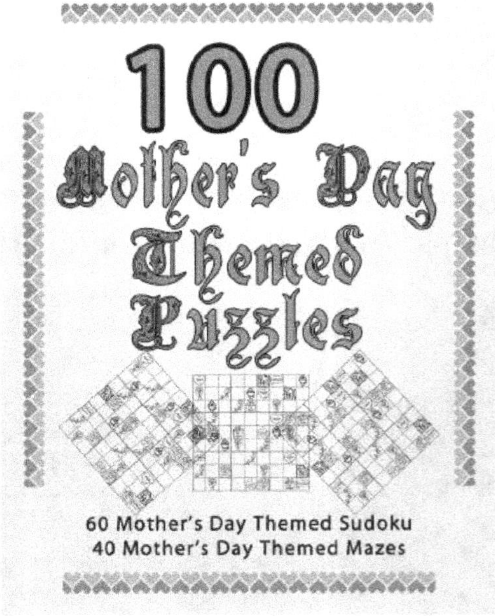

Want Even MORE Puzzle fun?
Try These Holiday Themed Puzzles!

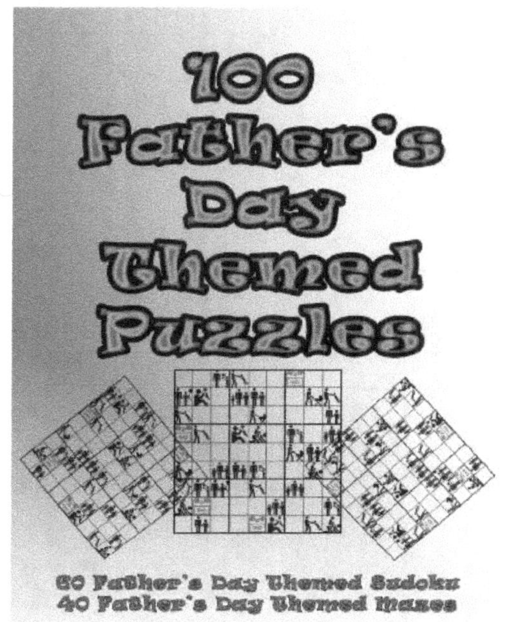

Father's Day Themed Puzzles
https://www.amazon.com/dp/1698823592

4th Of July Themed Puzzles
https://www.amazon.com/dp/169928539X

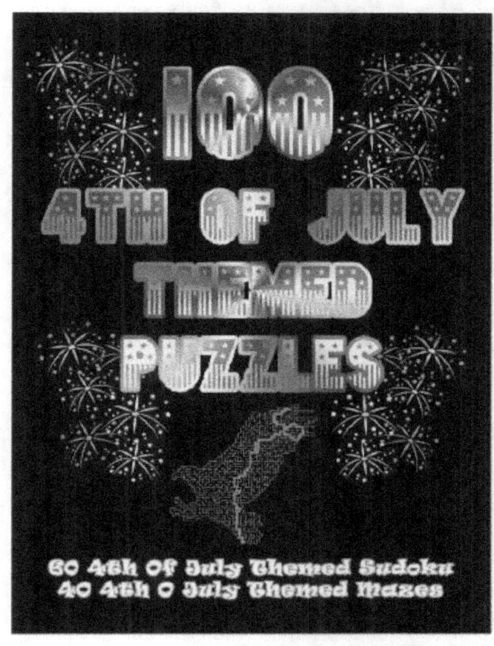

www.ingramcontent.com/pod-product-compliance
Lightning Source LLC
Chambersburg PA
CBHW081613250726
48657CB00009B/2561